Quality, risk
control in healt...

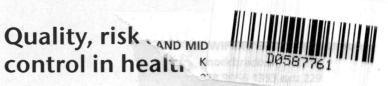

Quality, risk and control in health care

Ellie Scrivens

Open University Press

Open University Press
McGraw-Hill Education
McGraw-Hill House
Shoppenhangers Road
Maidenhead
Berkshire
England
SL6 2QL

email: enquiries@openup.co.uk
world wide web: www.openup.co.uk

and Two Penn Plaza, New York, NY 10121-2289, USA

First published 2005

A catalogue record of this book is available from the British Library

ISBN 0 335 20711 1 (pb)   0 335 20712 X (hb)

Library of Congress Cataloguing-in-Publication Data
CIP data applied for

Typeset by RefineCatch Limited, Bungay, Suffolk
Printed in the UK by MPG Books, Bodmin, Cornwall

Contents

For Justine, Kester, David and Gill

Foreword

At the heart of the debate about the delivery of health care in Britain – as in other countries – lies a fundamental challenge. Is it possible to devise a system of governance for the health care system which can reconcile seemingly contradictory policy objectives: the achievement of national policy objectives and standards of quality, on the one hand, and freedom for the managers and professionals responsible for delivery freedom to devise local solutions to local problems? How best can we strike a balance between regulatory over-kill and anarchic diversity, between protecting ourselves against risk and squeezing out innovation and exploration?

These are some of the concerns that shape Ellie Scrivens' book, an important contribution not only to the current debate about the NHS but also to the wider health care organisational literature. In it she explores some of the key issues involved. Most centrally, she addresses the question of how control over quality and performance should be exercised: whether any national system of external review should look at outputs, outcomes, processes, behaviour or the internal systems of control of the organisations being reviewed. Which in turn leads to a discussion of how standards should be written, of the role of inspectorates in enforcing them and of what the currency and lines of accountability should be.

All this is much-trawled ground, by myself among others (which is no doubt why I was asked to write this foreword). But the book also introduces and explores new dimensions. It explores the flow of ideas about governance from the private to the public sector. It documents the role and potentials of audit. It provides a history, informed by Professor Scrivens' own participation in the process, of the Department of Health's controls assurance programme designed to provide a governance structure for the boards of NHS trusts.

So the book passes what is my test for an interesting contribution to debate. It provides not only reassurance (Professor Scrivens has clearly read everything there is to be read) but also provides surprises (Professor Scrivens introduces a reader like myself to new ideas). While I am not sure that I share the author's commitments to notions of self-regulation based on risk assessment, I am quite sure that I will be able to argue about these and other questions in a much more informed way as a result of reading the book.

Rudolf Klein

Preface

For many years there has existed a popular view that management is unnecessary in health care. Doctors and nurses left to their own devices are able to provide the best health care. However, there is no universal agreement on the definition of 'best'. In our western-style democratic society, we are concerned equally with ensuring that decisions are taken in ways that conform to our values which, in turn, defines what we mean by good treatment. Recent events such as the retention of children's organs at Alder Hey Hospital demonstrate that doctors and other health care professionals may not share public values about what is perceived as good practice. Therefore, in order to address our concerns about what we mean by best health care, we have to address not only issues of clinical practice but also the issues of governance, decision making and better management processes – to ensure the organizations are able to deliver what we are asking of them. In short, we are seeking a process of 'New Governance', which will enable us to receive health care in the way we want it, putting our values – as patient and funder of health care – at the centre of decision making in health care.

The ideas underpinning New Governance in health services have their genesis in a number of different areas. It has long been recognized that any producer or employer can, through their production processes, cause harm to their staff, customers or society at large. Health services are as open to criticism as any organization that they can create pollution, or that they can damage staff through accidents. Protection from pollution and harm to staff are provided for in legislation, which applies as much to health care organizations as it does to any other employer or producer. Boards of NHS organizations are expected to follow legal requirements to ensure they are good employers and protectors of their local communities. Health care organizations deal with large amounts of public money, and are expected to protect themselves against risk of fraud and impropriety. Health care organizations are expected to deliver on government's promises to provide improved health care delivery, which requires a broader and more strategic assessment of risk associated with the management of their organizations. In addition, health care organizations face some specific risks. The very nature of health care means that patients can be put at risk by health care interventions and the risks associated with these are now recognized and health services are expected to deal with them. Almost every activity provided by a health care organization or its staff in dealing with the public entails a risk to patient health and safety, and health care managers are required to ensure that patients are afforded protection from harm wherever possible.

It was not until the 1970s that quality became applied to health care – often as an antidote to the overpowering emphasis on cost reduction and efficiency. All health care systems can spend more money than is made available to them. Advances in technology and people's desire for higher and higher quality of life have meant that there will always be more demand for health care than can be afforded. As health care systems expanded to cover more demand, pressures arose to reduce the expenditure on individual clinical procedures. There was a growing emphasis on cost reduction, creating a perceived trade-off between cost and quality of services. In addition, new technologies require increasing numbers of highly skilled people which, in turn, increases the complexity of the task of the management of health care, thus requiring new management skills. Hospitals with hundreds of beds employ thousands of people, to make sure that patients are well cared for. These range from doctors and nurses and people with other clinical skills, all increasingly highly trained and specialized to use the sophisticated equipment available; catering staff to make sure food is provided properly to help healing and health; cleaners to ensure a clean environment; estate managers to keep the buildings and equipment in proper order; and many others. Health care systems may spend over 70 per cent of their income on staff. Every patient uses the services of large numbers of people from doctors and nurses, to cleaners, porters, managers and finance experts. Ensuring that every one of these people is able to contribute to a service that is not only what patients want, but in a way that matches the personal and professional aspirations of staff, is a challenging task.

Between 2000 and 2004 I have had the privilege of being the Director of the Controls Assurance Support Unit, tasked with the role of supporting the NHS to introduce a standardized system of internal control across all NHS organizations. This was a unique opportunity to take part in a national experiment of vast scale. The NHS employs nearly one million people and uses over 800 organizations to deliver health care to the population of England. It is a national organization which has to provide care of an equivalent quality to each person who uses it and co-ordinate all the necessary organizational functions to ensure each individual receives the best possible care. Part of my role was to evaluate the impact of the controls assurance project. As a Professor of Health Policy, I found it necessary to review the origins of the concept of controls assurance and to place it in the wider context of developments taking place in the regulation of private businesses. I had to review developments in the professions of internal and external audit and also to examine recent government policy which influenced the development of controls assurance. I wanted to place controls assurance in the context of the wider developments taking place in the running not only of health services, but of central government, particularly the growing emphasis on devolution of power to local organizations. The government had decentralized power to a large number of independent agencies which, rather than improving the quality of health care or reducing bureaucracy were, in my opinion, doing little for quality and escalating bureaucracy. This book is the product of this extensive review.

In trying to explain the history and the recent policy developments, I have been forced to review a large number of documents. I was struck by the significance of many of these in developing the current views about governance in organizations and its relationship with internal control. I wanted to convey the significance of these writings to the current structures and policies. Therefore, I have included quotations to demonstrate the inter-relationship between these ideas which I hope, in the context of this topic, enhance rather than detract from the story.

However, the analysis revealed, as did my own personal experience, that although the controls assurance initiative introduced by the Department of Health was far ahead of its time in recognizing the need for a standardized approach to internal control, which would provide much needed public accountability for the actions of organizations, the approach was complicated and made more so by the array of different central initiatives to control the NHS. The introduction of the policy-creating, independent Foundation Trusts, believed to be fundamental to the improvement of quality and the progress of modernizing the National Health Service, would be seriously undermined if the confusion at the centre about the nature and the purpose of controls were not removed. In 2004, the unit of which I am Director changed its name to the Health Care Standards support unit, to provide support to the new Department of Health initiative on standards. I believe, based on my own research into the impact of standards on health care, that the recent emphasis on standards is an opportunity to develop further accountability for the quality of health care.

This book examines the arguments, debates and decisions that have been taken to create the governance infrastructure which allows these new developments to occur. It is predominantly concerned with the UK experience, as the UK has always had its own approach to the governance of business and this has impacted on assumptions about the governance of public sector services. In addition, due to the period of time upon which the subject matter focuses, this book is also a review of government policy at the turn of the twenty-first century. In some respects, the UK has been a pathfinder for other countries in that its experience of managing a national health service, and its approach to regulating private business have provided different models from those adopted in other countries. This book examines the changes that have been occurring in central government and local health care management resulting in the opportunity for 'New Governance' to occur. The book examines the issues in controlling the provision of health care and the new opportunities for thinking about the monitoring and management of health services. To do this it has been necessary to examine the arguments for changing our approach to the provision of health care and to ascertain how we want to manage health care in the new millennium.

Chapter One provides a brief review of the dimensions of quality that form the basic elements of quality needed to assure the public that health services are meeting their expectations. It is based upon a lecture I gave in Cork at the invitation of the Office for Health Management in Ireland which from 2005 will be part of the Health Service Executive in Ireland. I am grateful to them for the opportunity to develop my thinking in this area. Chapter Two reviews issues in the provision of assurance and the relationship between risk and control that has emerged from the corporate governance literature. This is central to the development of assurance under the government policy of devolved management. A related component in the provision of assurance is the building of public trust in public services and, therefore, the relationship of trust to accountability is also examined. Different approaches to describing control are developed as a framework for examining the approaches to assurance and control, and the views of corporate governance that have emerged in the private sector and central government departments. Chapter Three examines the emergence of risk and control as central issues in the development of governance in the private sector, along with ideas of increased stakeholder involvement in the production of accountability. Chapter Four examines how ideas about regulation by central governments have changed and how the ideas of corporate governance from the private sector have been translated into central government for use in civil service departments. Chapter Five examines how the limitations of regulation, inspection and audit in the NHS have led to the further development of ideas about the need for improved corporate governance in the NHS, and how these, in turn, have led to the concept of standardizing controls across the national health service. Chapter Six examines the arguments for change in the present accountability and assurance arrangements (particularly considering the limitations of current models of audit and inspection) and develops the argument for a new model. Chapter Seven concludes with the arguments for a new model of governance to meet the specific needs generated by the desire to provide assurance on quality in health care under a policy of devolving management to individual health care organisations.

The conclusion of the book is that a multidimensional model of assurance is needed to deliver public accountability in health care in a devolved management system, which has to have as its main focus improving the trust of the public in the health services that exist to serve them. And I must point out that the views and any errors in this book are wholly my responsibility and are not those of the Department of Health.

Ellie Scrivens
Health Care Standards Unit
Keele University
June 2004

Acknowledgements

I should like to thank the very many people who have helped me to understand the complex issues now developing in the field of governance and internal control in health care. There are too many to list them individually. Almost everyone I have spoken to over the past four years has contributed to my thinking and understanding. But there are a few special thanks I should like to make. I am deeply indebted to the team at the Health Care Standards Unit, previously known as the Controls Assurance Support Unit. Mrs Kim Donovan started out this voyage of exploration with me as we puzzled our way through the changes in government policy. Dr Katherine Birch has helped to shed light on the developments in risk management in the NHS. Mrs Janice Goldstraw, Dr Kate Wilde and Mrs Sue Fawcett have helped me in the understanding of the impact of controls assurance and standards on the NHS. Mr Phil O'Rourke has been invaluable in providing technical input without which I could not have worked my way through the ever growing body of literature on risk and governance. And I should like to thank Mrs Hazel Swift, Miss Helen Newton and Mrs Pat Leadbeater who provided moral support and organized me.

I should also like to thank Mr Robert May from the Department of Health who first introduced me to controls assurance and the ideas underpinning it. His vision for controls assurance provided the opportunity to pilot an approach to standardizing approaches to risk management, in order to deliver improved accountability. More recently, I have worked with Mr Stephen Mackenney and Dr Paul Stanton from the Clinical Governance Support Unit who have provided me with insights into clinical governance and the workings of the Department of Health. I am also grateful to Mr Chris Butler of the Treasury Risk Support Unit who has helped me to understand the development of risk management in government policy. Any mistakes I have made in the explanation of the development of risk management in central government and other areas are entirely mine. The Audit Commission and the National Audit Office also provided me with ideas and insights and to them I am grateful.

But most of all, I should like to thank David Rogers and my two children Kester and Justine, whose patience and tolerance in dealing with the chaos ensuing from the documents used in writing this book has been endless. And I apologize to Justine who wanted more pictures and larger letters so she and other little children could read it.

Ellie Scrivens
Keele
June 2004

1 The search for good quality health care: establishing principles for control

Health services across the world are being reinvented. The National Health Service in England has embarked upon a massive set of changes, moving from a state run, highly bureaucratic system to one intended to be more innovative and more concerned about improving patient care. On 15 January 2002 the then Secretary of State, Alan Milburn, pronounced a new vision for the National Health Service.

> What we envisage is a fundamentally different sort of NHS. Not a state run structure, but a values based system, where greater diversity and devolution are underpinned by common standards and a common public service ethos.
>
> (Rt Hon Alan Milburn MP 2002)

This statement suggests a vision of a more organic health care system, based upon common values and recognized standards, which will permit diversity in its management and design while recognizing a central core of best clinical practice and a public service ethos. The challenge, therefore, is to move from a highly centralized system, which dictates an identical structure and functioning of all the organizations that make up the national health service, to a more organic health care system, which is able to adapt its structure and its processes to meet local and individual needs while at the same time recognizing common definitions of good quality and good clinical care.

This requires a change in thinking about the management of health care and changes in the way health services are run. There is a need to establish a new system of governance for health care that enables care to be delivered in ways that are meaningful to patients and to the public who pay for them. The main objective of health care is to achieve health outcomes, better health and wellbeing for individuals. However, it is generally agreed that to demonstrate that outcomes are achieved requires measurement, and methods of measurement are elusive, at least at present. Therefore, there has been a tendency for health care organizations, and the governments who seek to control them, to look for processes that can be specified and to control the actions of the people who deliver health care. Quality is, therefore, frequently defined not in terms of the health of the patient, but in terms of the processes that contribute to care. The reliance on processes is not of itself a bad thing. Good processes are necessary to ensure that the right things happen, that the right drugs are given at the right time, that patients receive the right operation. Health care depends upon many complex processes which if wrongly undertaken, can result in unintended and often disastrous outcomes (Rt Hon Alan Milburn MP 2002). As a consequence the control of the people who administer care to patients became, in the past, the pre-occupation of those who control the quality of health care.

However, central control has not provided the incentives for innovation and the focus upon the patient (patient-centredness) that are required by modern patients and health care systems. The new values reflect more diverse and complex attitudes to quality, seeking to address the expectations of patients and the public rather than the expectations of those who provide health care. There is, therefore, a need to find new governance processes which can reflect these changed expectations for health care and ensure health services conform to wider societal expectations of the role of health services.

Health care has always been a major love of populations – it is not only the means to good health and long life, it is a symbol of democratic rights and citizenship, therefore, no-one should be denied the right to health and to a good quality of life. But this definition of access is relatively new. Beveridge, in outlining his social security plans for Britain post the Second World War, placed great emphasis on the need for a comprehensive health service (Sir William Beveridge 1942). Prevention was a key issue, though not for the reason often given today (i.e. the right to quality of life) but in order to afford the social security system he so desired.

> It is a logical corollary to the payment of high benefits in disability that determined efforts should be made by the State to reduce the number of cases for which benefit is needed. It is a logical corollary to the receipt of high benefit in disability that the individual should recognize the duty to be well and to cooperate in all steps which lead to the diagnosis of disease in early stages when it can be prevented.
>
> (Sir William Beveridge 1942 Para 426)

Today, satisfaction (particularly with regard to waiting times) with health care services is seen as an important indicator of how well a health care system serves its population. Long waiting lists have been thought to be the reason for an apparently high level of dissatisfaction and have been used to justify not only a governmental policy emphasis on reducing waiting times but also the need for better understanding of the whole system and how patients move through the health care process (Houses of the Oireachtais 2002).

Beveridge was concerned that 'suitable hospital treatment [should be] available for every citizen and that recourse to it, at the earliest moment when it becomes desirable, is not delayed by any financial consideration' (Sir William Beveridge 1942). Today, delay in any shape or form is a prime consideration of access to health care. Equally, there is an awareness that different ethnic or social groups may have different experiences of health care through unconscious discrimination, and health systems are becoming aware of the need to address these issues. The approach to this varies as the impact of discrimination varies in different countries. In the United States, 42.6 million Americans are estimated to lack health insurance, many of whom are in racial and ethnic minorities (Health Resources and Services Administration 2000). In the UK, there is concern that religious practices may be overlooked by professionals who fail to appreciate the impact of these upon the ability of patients to use or gain benefit from health care (Department of Health 2000).

A second aspect of access is ensuring that everyone who needs health care gets the right services. This requires that special services are provided to meet the needs of particular groups in society. And recently, a third aspect has also become important. One of the major changes in our thinking about quality of health care came from an understanding that people's willingness to use health care depends upon their relationship with the health care system. Avedis Donabedian, the father of the concept of quality in health care, also included accessibility to be a highly subjective attribute. He felt that accessibility of care, the doctor-patient relationship and the 'amenities of care' greatly influence acceptability, legitimacy and equity in health services (Donabedian 1990). Therefore, when thinking about equity and fairness, we have to consider what is acceptable to people in terms of their personal value systems and their personal desires, as well as what might be considered, in objective terms, good for them.

Beveridge and indeed most commentators and social reformers of his time were not concerned with variability in clinical practice. Only relatively recently have differences been recognized, not only in the way that services are experienced by patients but also in the way they are delivered by individual clinicians and in the differential use of resources in treating conditions. These may be attributable to individual doctors having access to different training and information but differences in the management of waiting lists and other key indicators of access to health care have also been identified. It is postulated that something more complex than simply the differential skills of clinicians is causing the level of variation. Variations in the quality of health care are evident from studies, even in systems such as the NHS, which are intended to have (through high levels of central control) the same basic administrative, resource allocation and management approaches.

Safety

If Governments are charged with protecting the public from risks caused by the direct provision of services, governments face a duty to ensure that the risks to the public using the services are minimized. Modern health care presents the most complex challenge in terms of safety of any activity on earth (Leape *et al.* 1998). Harmful or adverse events have been reported for many years (since the 1950s and 1960s). Research in the USA, Australia and the UK has demonstrated the seriousness and the high levels of health care induced harm (an adverse event rate of 3.8–5.4 per cent in hospital admissions in the USA; 10.6, 16.6 per cent in Australia, 11.7 per cent in the UK and 9.0 per cent in Denmark) and has brought safety to the forefront of national and international thinking on quality (World Health Organisation Secretariat 2001). Medical errors are now considered to be unacceptable and have only recently been the subject of public and policy attention. Research in the USA suggests that of the over 33.6 million admissions to US hospitals in 1997 that 44,000 and possibly as many as 98,000 Americans died and will die each year, as a result of medical errors (Kohn, Corrigan and Donaldson 2000). This led the authors of the Institute of Medicine report, *To Err is Human*, to conclude that more people die in a given year as a result of medical errors than from motor vehicle accidents or breast cancer. One study estimated that the average intensive care unit patient in the USA experienced almost two errors a day. This caused the authors of the study to point out that a performance level of 99.9 per cent (higher than that experienced in intensive care units) applied to the airline and banking industries would equate to two dangerous landings at O'Hare international airport and 32,000 cheques deducted from the wrong bank account per hour (Leape 1994).

This concern caused the UK, the USA and Australia, as well as others, to focus on the need to improve national commitment to safety and quality, and to co-ordinate quality activities. The UK government introduced a ten-year plan to refocus the National Health Service and the USA began to develop a national co-ordinated approach to quality measurement and reporting (National Expert Advisory Group on safety and quality in Australian health care 1999). Many countries, including the UK, established national systems to record and document the causes of medical errors in an attempt to identify the root causes of these and, where possible, to introduce systems and preventive measures to eradicate them (Department of Health 2001a). There was much talk of the need to change the culture of health care services to what was termed a 'safety culture', in which staff are encouraged to report incidents and what are termed 'near misses', to enable learning to occur which will prevent the situations from being repeated. In addition, patients are actively encouraged to participate in health care, and to not just assume that they will receive appropriate and safe care (Gaba 2000; Roberts 1990).

The total national cost of preventable adverse events in the USA was estimated at between $17 000 and 29 000 million US dollars a year. In the UK, the estimate was about £2000 million a year plus £2400 million in potential liability for negligence claims and £1000 million for hospital acquired infection. And as the WHO points out 'added to these costs is the erosion of trust, confidence and satisfaction amongst the public and health care providers' (World Health Organisation Secretariat 2001).

Efficiency and effectiveness

In the 1960s and 1970s, when quality started to creep into discussions of health care, there was a belief that quality should be modelled upon industrial or manufacturing concepts of quality. This suggested that quality could be specified in advance and by following recipes for quality production, health care quality could be guaranteed. Some two decades ago a distinction was drawn between what has become called technical quality and functional quality (Gronroos 1984). Functional quality is how the patient receives a service, for example, the quality of nurse/patient interaction and the condition of the environment. Measures of patient satisfaction with hospital care have focused on the quality of food, the condition of the surroundings and so on. But although these are important in terms of providing patient comfort, they do not address the issue of the content of the clinical care provided – the technical aspects of the quality of health care delivery.

Technical quality is described as the material content during the buyer-seller interaction of what the customer receives – the technical aspects of clinical care – which equates to competence (professional expertise qualifications) and patient outcomes (rate of cure, mortality rates). Evidence suggests that physicians still tend to identify quality using these dimensions. They define outcomes as minimizing/curing disease and/or rate of cure (Jun, Peterson and Zsidisin 1998). However, it is thought by many involved in health care evaluation that this aspect of health care quality exceeds the full understanding of most patients. Without technical training, how can a patient judge whether a clinician did a good job? Excellence in technical quality is the attainment of the best possible clinical outcome. But this does not reflect the other aspects of quality of health care which patients might be expected to be concerned with such as the ability to regain functioning after a health care encounter or quality of life. This view also does not take into account the cost effectiveness or appropriateness of different sorts of treatment. A major question facing all health care systems is how best to organize health care to achieve consistently, and across all parts, the best outcome affordable for the resources available.

Systems theory

Donabedian (1980) drew attention to systems in health care and the importance of thinking about health care as a system with structure, processes and
outputs, which changed thinking about quality in two ways (Donabedian
1988b). First, Donabedian's ideas enabled health care to be viewed as provided
by a number of interlocking organizations rather than as a collection of
independent organizations, such as hospitals and clinics. It became necessary
to analyse the ways in which patients pass through a number of different
organizations, from primary health care to secondary and tertiary care, and
maybe terminal care, in their receipt of health care. Second, these ideas began
the much more difficult process of thinking about the management of change
in an industry that is subject to continuous and rapid change.

Any change will have consequences for a system, therefore, in an industry
that is constantly changing through innovation, new technologies and new
drugs, there is a need to review continuously the impact of changes. This has
been described as a 'beyond blame culture' which emphasizes the value of
systems, supported by processes and frameworks for identifying, evaluating
and implementing system-based approaches to safety and quality. This is
analogous to the processes and frameworks used in the airline industry
(National Expert Advisory Group on safety and quality in Australian health
care 1999). Those working within the system need to be aware of 'things going
wrong' or 'not achieving what is required'. It is beginning to be recognized
that it is possible to over-engineer systems. For example, in the market for
software, most products are capable of doing more than most consumers
require and never use. There are too many safeguards to ensure that mistakes
do not occur and because of this the software does not deliver the speed or the
ease of use that consumers would require. In health care routine, yet important, work processes may have 30 or 40 steps and involve people from five or six
departments and clinical disciplines. Because no individual knows all the
steps, there are often redundant and unnecessary processes which create
delays in the delivery of care.

The specification of processes has led to a growing emphasis on pre-agreed
standards and organizational processes. However, health care workers and
politicians frequently complain about the burdens of bureaucracy introduced
in the over-engineering of the systems. But in many cases, patients rely on
bureaucracy to protect them. In health care, learning from mistakes is necessary but for individual patients there is no chance to undo disastrous consequences of actions. Learning from experience is often bought at the high
price of human suffering and possibly death. There are, therefore, some
areas where health care needs to be over-engineered and highly structured,
such as in the prevention of health care acquired infections. In the UK, in

February 2000, the National Audit Office suggested that hospital acquired infections were estimated to cost the NHS £1billion per year and led to the deaths of as many as 5,000 patients (Taylor, Plowman and Roberts 2001). Improving quality in health care requires a better balance between prescription of necessary actions and trust of professional staff to do the right thing. Management systems need to be designed to help clinicians to ensure their practice is safe and effective without introducing burdensome regulatory and monitoring systems (Halligan and Donaldson 2001).

Managing systems – leadership

Leadership is important in systems. Different departments, people, equipment, facilities and functions make up an organization. A leader's job is to integrate these diverse components so they accomplish the common purpose (Kouzes and Posner 1999). They do this by setting clear objectives for the organization and creating a framework for accountability for decisions and performance (Audit Commission 2003: 39). For a long time it was believed that leaders are born rather than created but it now thought that leadership is an observable, learnable set of practices. Modern leadership, particularly that provided in health care teams, is no longer based upon hierarchical management. Teams can solve problems much better than individuals and research has shown that a team will find ways to solve problems more quickly than formal education can achieve, providing they have some basic understanding of what they are trying to achieve (Mitra and Rana 1999). However, if the team is too big, there is evidence that this will slow down the problem-solving process. Health care management has to recognize the significance of ensuring the right size and composition of teams, to manage change continuously and address the new risks that are continually presented in health care.

There has been a slow recognition of the idea that for systems improvements to be developed, approaches based on an embedded planning cycle of plan, do, check, then act, are better than experimental designs (Brennan and Berwick 1995: 351). That is, pragmatic management through action is better than waiting for long-term experimentation to produce the right results. Health care systems have, in recognizing these issues, embraced what has been called the principle of continuous quality improvement. This is a theory of management, introduced in the 1960s, which health care organizations toyed with for many years but did not wholly embrace. But as health care organizations have accepted the importance of systems, so they have also begun to implement the ideas of continuous quality improvement. One main proponent of this idea, Deming, provides an insight into what managers need to understand.

Deming's management theory is derived from an application of what he calls a system of profound knowledge (Deming 2002). This requires an understanding of the psychology of customers, how variations in the system can be identified and measured, and a theory of knowledge about how the system works. Deming estimated that 85 per cent of corporate failures arise from bad systems not bad workers (Lea and Mayo 2002: 3). Complex systems require continuous analysis to understand their operations and to ensure fairness and accountability. In 1979, Williamson and his colleagues estimated that less than 20 per cent of common medical process of care factors had any scientific basis established through clinical research (Williamson, Goldschmidt and Jilson 1979). This figure is less now as the clinical professions have begun to apply an approach called 'evidence-based medicine', collecting together all the available evidence to assess what is really known about a drug, treatment or procedure.

> Real improvement in quality depends, according the Theory of Continuous Improvement on understanding and revising the production processes on the basis of data about the processes themselves. The focus is on continuous improvement through constant effort to reduce waste, rework and complexity.
>
> (Berwick 1989: 54)

Clinicians are also expected to monitor their own experiences of providing care through clinical audit and review programmes. However, they cannot assess the impact of the whole system on their work. It is being realized that it is the task of health care management to provide the data analysis support to clinicians, to allow them to understand what they should do.

The emphasis on systems has also revealed a new proposition. Health care is not just one single integrated system but consists of a large number of inter-related systems, which are involved in the provision of health care: the multiplicity of small organizational systems, which are needed to admit patients, generate and keep records, ensure communications are established; the clinical systems, which provide diagnoses, enable operating theatres to run; and the patient who is a system in their own right with their own inputs in terms of physiology and psychology, their adaptability to treatment programmes and processes and their own outputs in terms of physical functioning, quality of life and satisfaction with the whole experience of consuming health care. All these separate parts have to be managed to achieve the objectives of each individual system, and these objectives have to be aligned to ensure they are compatible with each other, to produce a total, integrated health care system.

It is also the case that errors occur in complex systems through the concatenation of multiple small failures, which individually produce vulnerabilities in the systems and, when activated at the same time, can produce catastrophic failure. However, properly constituted teams and systems are able to recognize trouble before problems arise (Leape *et al.* 1998). Flexible project teams must be created, trained and competently led to tackle complex processes that cross the customary departmental boundaries. And this is where accountability structures become important in the quest for quality. People have to understand their contribution to the whole system of care and to value their place within the system, understanding who is responsible for the provision of care, who is responsible for identifying when changes create risk in the system and who is responsible for addressing those risks is fundamental to improving quality in health care.

Teamwork requires collaboration of all the people working within a system. 'Concepts of teamwork and the synergistic effect of various actors in providing health care "commingling" of all the roles of all members of the health care team including payers, physicians, patients, family members and members of the community' (Jun, Peterson and Zsidisin 1998). This emphasizes the importance of communication for successful collaboration. Communication fills the gaps to prevent disjointed service between patients and clinicians, between clinical colleagues, between clinicians and other staff working in the same organization, and between different organizations. All team members need to understand what part they play in achieving the objectives.

Patient-centred approaches

To enable individuals to achieve their full health potential, there is a need to move to a more relevant set of assumptions about the role of the patient in considering the quality of health care. This should be done through a search for appropriate and relevant judgements that consumers of services can and do use to assess quality (Donabedian 1990). In many studies of service quality across different sectors, from banking to getting a television repaired, researchers have been surprised to find that consumers have different perceptions of the parameters of quality from those who provide the service. Bankers think their job is about keeping money secure – customers think the job of a bank is to help them get access to their money when they want it, quickly and helpfully. When automatic teller machines were introduced 20 years ago, the banking industry was surprised about how many people would prefer to stand in the rain waiting in a queue to get to the machine, rather than go into the bank to deal with a human teller. In addition, it is being recognized that patients can see more of the totality of the system than anyone working in just a part of it. The patient travels through the whole process and can observe the whole organization. Health care organizations and systems need to listen to what patients say about the experience in order to learn and to improve and to ensure that their views are taken into account.

Equally, a study in the UK of quality priorities for elderly patients demonstrated that the key difference between professionals and patients occurred in the importance attached to reducing the burden on family care-givers. Patients saw this as a priority whereas professionals were more concerned about physical functioning (Roberts and Philip 1996). Swedish researchers found that significant predictors of quality ratings included information concerning one's illness – that is, it is very important to provide information to patients about the care that they will receive and the whole experience of being a patient (Arnetz and Arnetz 1996). Studies in the USA have shown that total quality management in health care starts from educating the patient in how to get the best from the health care system. Indeed, various patient support organizations in the USA have now produced documents for patients advising them that they are responsible for ensuring that they are treated safely, as well as giving them advice on how to ensure they are receiving the right care that they require. It is believed that health care systems have to ensure patients have their say, are listened to and their views are taken fully into account when planning both individual care and health systems.

Quality has to be treated as more akin to an attitude, made up of many different influences on patient and public perceptions. It is particularly important in health care because perceptions of health care and health care providers can have a strong impact upon our overall health behaviours. Compliance with behavioural requirements, such as taking prescribed drugs, is something that patients do not do readily. Research has discovered that to obtain the necessary compliance to improve health, health services have to deal with the whole patient if they are to achieve the intended outcomes and must recognize that their attitude to patients and the caring provided contributes to the self-image and esteem patients award to themselves. This impacts on the compliance of patients as high self-worth improves the likelihood of compliance (Montgomery 1993).

Quality of care also requires that clinicians recognize and understand the need for continuous reflection upon their relationships with patients and the ability to learn from their practice and any errors made, in order to continually improve the services they are providing. Are the checks in place that ensure the patient is safe? This includes ensuring that doctors are well trained in clinical procedures and knowledge; they have systems in place to check they have done things properly; they understand their roles and responsibilities in the system for providing health care; and they monitor their own performance in order to assess where they need help to improve (Halligan and Donaldson 2001; Scally and Donaldson 1998). The quality of health care, therefore, relates directly to public perceptions of trust in those who deliver health services.

Quality is also determined by the appropriate use of resources. There is a need to know whether particular treatments provide benefit for the resources used. No clinician, doctor, nurse or other health care professional operates in isolation. They are part of a complex system involving many different people and many different actions but they can each individually distort the system or prevent it from operating effectively, if they do not, themselves, operate effectively and efficiently. Expensive treatments can be used for the benefit of a few at the expense of providing other services for the many. Unrestricted choice of the use of resources by individual doctors may lead to resources going to groups of patients, contradictory to the wishes of society in general. These are never easy decisions, and they reflect the continuing tension between the clinical desire to do the best for patients balanced against the health care needs of the whole population. Therefore, considerations of quality must also take into account how decisions on health care resources are made. Public perceptions of quality, therefore, need to influence resource allocation decisions and to ensure that health care reflects the preferences and wishes of the community served by the health care system. Communities need to shape the inputs of the programmes to decide where the money is best spent. Different approaches have been tried to use community views to influence the ways in which resource allocation decisions are made. The Oregon experiments, which attempted to use public opinion to set health care priorities, or the involvement of local politicians in the health care resource allocation process are examples of ways in which this has been approached (Hadorn 1991).

The focus on the patient emphasizes a number of dimensions of quality that are central to the patient's experience of health care: safety, in terms of reducing risks of interventions and in the environment; efficiency, where the results of care and interventions are related to resources used; respect and caring, which demonstrates the degree to which the patient or designee is involved in their own care decisions and the degree to which those providing services do so with sensitivity and respect for the patient's needs, expectations and individual differences.

Service quality is judged by consumers according to a number of cues relating to the delivery of the service and personal experience. Patients also are thought to use similar cues to evaluate the quality of health care. For example, Baker and Pink identify a number of dimensions:

- Time – did the patient receive the service promptly?
- Process quality – was the service provided free of error?
- Service – was the service provided in a comfortable and respectful manner?
- Outcome – did the service alleviate the patient's problem?
- Cost – was the service provided in such as way as to minimize cost and inconvenience to the patient and family?

(Baker and Pink 1995)

An essential part of health care quality improvement becomes the patient's ability to access information on outcomes of treatments, patient personal assessments of quality of care and other quality indicators. As Eisenberg has pointed out:

> . . . if I am buying a car, I know that I can find data on the safety, efficiency, and reliability of different car models. This data is based on accepted measurements, such as crash tests, service records and fuel efficiency. Like the automobile industry, we must make the goal of our health care system to provide similar information on the quality of health care services. To that end, we must strive to develop accepted measures and instruments used to gauge and improve the quality of health services.
>
> (Eisenberg 1997)

However, the judgement of quality is thought also to involve a comparison of expectations with performance. In the 1980s, a research project identified that gaps between what managers expected to provide and what consumers expected to receive leading to the proposition that 'the quality a consumer perceives in a service is a function of the magnitude and direction of the gap between expected service and perceived service' (Parasuraman, Zeithamel and Berry 1985: 46). Consumers are more likely to perceive service quality to be deteriorating when their expectations are not met in terms of their direct experience. And this leads to a reduction in satisfaction with the service provided. As public expectations of health care increase, so it becomes increasingly important to ensure that the direct experience of services matches expectations. Otherwise public dissatisfaction with services will continue to grow. One way to ensure patients' individual expectations are met is to empower patients to be actively involved in their care and treatment and to be able to choose between alternative forms of provision, thus defining their own expectations of care.

Public accountability

The definition of appropriate and responsive health care delivery cannot be divorced from patients' views. However, health services are also social institutions and cannot be divorced from wider societal views about how health care resources should be used (Day and Klein 1987; Klein and Day 1989). For health services to be held accountable for their actions, the parameters of what is meant by good health care nationally (and now internationally) have to be defined and agreed not only by those providing health care recognizing patients' preferences, but by all the societal stakeholders in the business of running health services. This requires health care organizations to be prepared to accept the advice, support and judgement of stakeholders in how services should be provided, managed and improved. But just as importantly, there has to be assurance that the people who work in health care services as well as the patients who use them, conform to expected behaviours in order to ensure that quality services are delivered in the way that is expected of them. The way this is accomplished is through the establishment and implementation of methods of controlling organizational and professional behaviour to ensure organizations comply with the required societal norms and legislative requirements placed upon them. There are many different ways in which health services are controlled by society, through central government regulations, through local political processes and through professionally determined norms of behaviour. Each health care system has a variety of approaches that have evolved to control the shape and the function of health services. But these approaches were developed at a time when the definition of health care was dominated by the views of professionals and central government. The new aspirations of modern society – emphasizing the centrality of patient choice and patient views of quality, and the desire to transfer decision making from the centre to local organizations – requires a new approach to the control of quality in health care.

Chapter summary

This chapter has dealt with the following points:

- The need for and definitions of quality in health care services.
- Safety, efficiency and effectiveness as quality factors.
- An overview of systems theory, and the management of a health care system.
- The need for patient-centred approaches, as well as public accountability, in providing a high quality health care service.

2   Controls and Assurance

The reduction in regulation

By the early 2000s, four major concerns began to preoccupy the UK government. These were:

1   the need for modernization, to improve the delivery of public services and to ensure public expectations for services were being met;
2   the need for devolved management to ensure that organizations could take advantage of freedom from the shackles of central control to innovate and thereby deliver, the desired modernization;
3   greater public accountability to ensure that the freer local organizations would be held democratically accountable for the innovation and modernizing actions they were to deliver;
4   these together would result in increased trust amongst the public towards the public services that exist on their behalf.

It was well recognized that public expectations for better public services had risen rapidly but policies had failed to produce a demonstrably better relationship between the public and the services which serve them. Rising standards of living, a more diverse society and a steadily stronger consumer culture were felt to have increased the demand for good quality public services.

It is the government's job to set national standards that really matter to the public within a clear framework of accountability desired to ensure that citizens have the right to high quality services wherever they live. These standards can only be delivered effectively by devolution and delegation to the front line, giving local leaders responsibility and accountability for delivery and the opportunity to design and develop services around the needs of local people. More flexibility is required for public service organisations and their staff to achieve the

Table 2.1 The government's principles of public service reform

- A national framework of standards and accountability.
- Devolution to the front-line, allowing far greater freedom and ro
so that local services develop as users want.
- Flexibility so that local organizations and their staff are better able to provide modern public services.
- More choice for the pupil, patient or consumer, and the ability if provision is poor to have an alternative provider.

(H.M. Treasury 2002b para 0.2)

diversity of service provision needed to respond to the wider range of customer aspirations. This means challenging restrictive practices and reducing red tape; greater and more flexible incentives and rewards for good performance; strong leadership and management; and high quality training and development. Public services need to offer expanding choice for the customer. Giving people a choice about the service they can have and who provides it helps to ensure that services are designed around their customers.

(The Prime Minister's Office of Public Services Reform 2002 page 10)

Greater choice, responsiveness, accessibility and flexibility were believed to be central to public expectations and these became the cornerstones of a new management agenda, which would allow organizations freedom to achieve these ends in the delivery of public services (The Prime Minister's Office of Public Services Reform 2002). In order to provide equity across the country, the government prescribed the use of national standards to which all devolved organizations would work, but the standards would have to provide for local diversity and flexibility in finding solutions to the modernization requirements. There was to be no national prescription for the form the services should take. Central government departments were felt to be unable to deliver this flexibility because they were unable to think creatively or strategically in innovating service design. Indeed, central government was thought to be guilty of actively preventing local innovation by the imposition of central regulation and bureaucracy (Strategic policy making team, Cabinet office 1999). It is, therefore, necessary that governments address how to reduce the amount of burdensome red tape placed upon organizations.

Governments have too often been ready to introduce new regulations, without removing old redundant ones. Clearly regulation has an important role in protecting the public, preventing fraud or ensuring minimum standards. But a key part of devolving power and

> responsibility will be the removal of needless bureaucratic rules. And
> if local managers are to be freer to innovate they need that freedom of
> movement which excess regulation can prevent.
> (The Prime Minister's Office of Public Services Reform 2002 page 19)

Modernization at all levels, therefore, necessitated radical changes to the
running of central government, which emphasized the need to change ideas of
public accountability and which were to have a direct impact upon how health
care will be managed. The first was change in the way the civil service – in the
case of health services, the Department of Health – controls the environment
in which businesses providing health care as well as the public sector services
operated. This required a reduction in the degree of regulation provided by
government. The second, following on from the first, was better and more
open decision making by government, which would inform the public of why
decisions were taken and involving them directly in decision taking. The third
was to be the reduction in central control over organizations which provided
public services and the introduction of greater local decision making to
achieve greater local accountability for the provision of services and to make
them more responsive to locally perceived needs.

Devolution of decision making was intended to lead to more flexible decision making, which would enable improvements in the delivery of services
through being better able to meet the expectations of service users. But to
maintain public accountability, new approaches to the delivery of more flexible services required a greater emphasis on local accountability, to ensure that
services were being provided appropriately and consistently across the country.
And this required a new understanding of governance as it relates not only to
central government as central control receded, but also to the workings of
locally run organizations as they strove to achieve improved service quality for
individual consumers.

> Greater delegation of responsibility will mean a greater risk of
> inconsistency. The public is rightly intolerant of this, with com-
> plaints of 'post code lotteries' in health care. There will need to be a
> counterbalancing increase in local accountability to allow local
> decisions to be scrutinized and justified.
> (Better regulation task force 2001 page 5)

In the public sector therefore, in line with the corporate governance
debate in the private sector, there were growing arguments for governance
arrangements for public services to strike the right balance between having the
freedom to innovate and achieve continuous improvement, and the need to
demonstrate accountability for and probity in the use of public monies (CIPFA/
SOLACE 2001). However, there had been attempts to introduce horizontal or

external decentralization as opposed to vertical/internal decentralisation (Yataganas 2001 page 7). Horizontal decentralization refers to the development of agencies to take over the functions of government. Between 1999 and 2004 aspects of work of the Department of Health were transferred to forty-two arms length bodies, established to reduce the work undertaken directly by central government and to be independent in their operation. These bodies were not set up with appropriate governance structures in many cases and, instead of encouraging innovation and change, became associated with a vast amount of bureaucracy and uncontrolled growth of prescription from the centre. Devolution, with its accent on the principles of partnership and subsidiarity is, therefore, a response designed to stem this tide of what has been described as 'regulatory and administrative bulimia.' (Yataganas 2001 page 5).

The search for new accountability

Accountability is being 'liable to be called to account', that is to explain one's actions to others and, by inference in this context, publicly. According to the Oxford English Dictionary, assurance is 'to tell a person confidently as a thing that he may trust'. Accountability is regarded as one of three pillars of democratic government, the others being the authority to govern, derived from the electoral process, and the ability of government to respond to the needs of all sections of society and not just its own constituents. For a government to be accountable for its actions it must clearly state its aims, its actions must be transparent and it must assume responsibility for the outcomes. If these conditions are not met, accountability is only partial (Scott 2000).

Under the principle of devolution, which requires changes in the responsibilities of central government for the delivery of public services, there must be greater accountability at a local level. For a local organization operating under limited control of central government to be properly accountable, its managers – that is, its boards or senior decision makers – must be able to be trusted to run the organization well. Accountability requires, therefore, that organizations and their management are willing and able to accept responsibility for their decisions and actions, including all aspects of performance, and submit themselves to appropriate external scrutiny. It is achieved by all parties having a clear understanding of those responsibilities, and having clearly defined roles within a robust structure (CIPFA/SOLACE 2001). For organizations that are owned by the government, the conditions of governmental accountability must combine with the requirements for organizational accountability.

The terms accountability and responsibility are frequently treated as separate concepts in the management literature. Managers, particularly in the public sector, are seen as responsible for delivering agreed actions, that is making sure things that should be done are being done within the organization (Treasury Board of Canada 1999). This applies to management as much as to organizational conduct. Responsibility is, therefore, often described as part of the internal delegation of management. Accountability, in contrast, is used to describe the process of ensuring that these responsibilities are fulfilled, explaining the outcomes of actions and decisions to the external world (Burgess, Burton and Parston 2001). The difference between the two concepts has been summarized as: 'corporate accountability requires independent oversight and enforcement mechanisms, whereas corporate responsibility relies on voluntary self-regulation' (Friends of the Earth 2001 page 1).

Accountability, therefore, involves both an upwards and an outwards thrust of assurance (see Figure 1), upwards to central government and outwards towards the local public and population served to ensure that individuals and organizations are first, able to demonstrate that organizational structures and processes are as expected and second, able to explain why decisions were taken and actions performed in the way that they were. Being held to account suggests that an organization is under some form of scrutiny for actions taken, either in the form of audit, inspection, inquiry by external assessors or performance monitoring by some superior body in the organizational hierarchy, not only when something has gone wrong but, more importantly, on routine daily activity to ensure that actions are conducted in line with societal and legal requirements. In the present situation, when central government is no longer considered capable of managing public services, and as a consequence, decision making is devolved to local organizations, the governance of local organizations becomes much more significant in the delivery of accountability to local publics. The local organizations must be able to

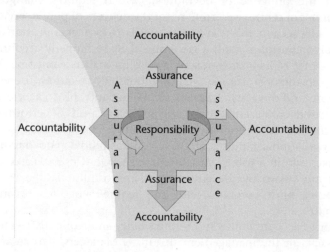

Figure 2.1   Accountability and assurance.

demonstrate the ability, and thereby be trusted, to control organizations and to manage risks that occur in the day-to-day running of their affairs, particularly those risks that derive from changing services and innovating to produce new methods of service delivery. Central government must be able to demonstrate the services are delivering against a national agenda, while also resisting the temptation to control local organizations.

Three inter-related concepts of trust, control and risk run as a leitmotif through this book. The theories of organizational management and governance described in this book are derived from assumptions about the relationships between these three concepts and how these together can deliver public accountability through governance. The development of the concepts of trust, control and risk have been determined by the development of accountability and governance.

Accountability, therefore, is a product of good governance, which is the way in which business corporations (later in this chapter applied to other governmental and related agencies) are directed and controlled. 'Corporate governance provides an architecture of accountability – structures and processes to ensure companies are managed in the interests of their owners' (Higgs 2003 page 11). The corporate governance structure specifies the distribution of rights and responsibilities among different interests in the business, including the board, managers, shareholders and other stakeholders. It also spells out the rules and procedures for making decisions on corporate affairs and in so doing, it provides the structure through which the company objectives are set, and the means of meeting those objectives and monitoring performance (OECD 2002). In public organizations, corporate governance also includes principles of conduct that should underpin the behaviour of public employees and their boards. These cover: selflessness, integrity, objectivity, accountability, openness, honesty and leadership (Committee on standards in public life 1996). In 2000, the government developed ten principles of conduct to apply to local government councillors and co-opted members in England. The principles follow those for central government, but in addition cover personal judgement, respect for others, duty to uphold the law and stewardship.

Corporate governance is, therefore, intended to secure and motivate the efficient management of companies and businesses, and can use mechanisms such as contracts, organizational design and legislation (encycogov.com 2004). The earliest definition of corporate governance is attributed to Milton Friedman. 'Corporate Governance is to conduct the business in accordance with owner or shareholders' desires, which generally will be to make as much money as possible, while conforming to the basic rules of the society embodied in law and local customs.' This definition is based on the economic concept of market value maximization that underpins shareholder capitalism. Over a period of time the definition of corporate governance has been widened and it now encompasses the interests of not only the shareholders but society at large, encompassing the need to consider many different groups of stakeholders (encycogov.com 2004).

It has been suggested that the origins of modern corporate governance are to be found in the Watergate scandal in the United States. As a result of subsequent investigations, US regulatory and legislative bodies were able to highlight failures in the systems that controlled the actions of major corporations, which had permitted them to make illegal political contributions and to bribe government officials. The response of the US government was to introduce the Foreign and Corrupt Practices Act 1977, which makes explicit reference to the establishment, maintenance and review of internal management systems – referred to as internal control. This was followed in 1979 by the Securities and Exchange Commission of USA's proposals for mandatory reporting on internal financial controls. In 1985, following a series of high-profile business failures in the USA, the most notable one of which being the Savings and Loan collapse, the Treadway Commission was formed (Treadway Report 1987). Its primary role was to identify the main causes of misrepresentation in financial reports and to recommend ways of reducing the incidence. The Treadway report (discussed in the next chapter), published in 1987, highlighted the need for a proper control environment, independent audit committees and an objective internal audit function. It also called for published reports on the effectiveness of internal control and requested the sponsoring organizations to develop an integrated set of internal control criteria to enable companies to improve their controls. The resulting committee, the Committee of Sponsoring Organizations (CoSo), produced a report in 1992, which described a framework of control (CoSo 1995).

There was similar experience of corporate failures and scandals in the UK, involving companies such as Polly Peck, British & Commonwealth, BCCI and Robert Maxwell's Mirror Group, which saw explosive growth in earnings, and all ended in disaster due to the poor management of business practices. These led to similar calls for improved corporate governance in the UK which, like developments in the USA, emphasized the need for improved internal control systems (OECD 2003). The Audit Commission has created its own definition of corporate governance for health care organizations that brings together the notion of accountability, leadership, control and objectives: 'The framework of accountability to users, stakeholders and the wider community, within which organisations take decisions, and lead and control their functions, to achieve their objectives' (Audit Commission 2003 page 4).

Control and control methods

Controls are the techniques used to produce desired behaviours. Control has been defined as 'a cybernetic, regulatory process that directs or constrains an interactive activity to some standard or purpose' (Green and Welsh 1998 page 291) or as 'a regulatory process by which the elements of a system are made more predictable through the establishment of standards in the pursuit of some desired objective or state' (Liefer and Mills 1996 page 117).

Governments use regulation – with sanctions attached to failure to comply with them – as controls designed to ensure citizens and organizations behave in socially desirable ways. To monitor appropriate behaviour of individuals, governments have a variety of methods available to them, such as policing and monitoring. To monitor the activities of organizations and their staff, governments can use visits and reviews by appointed inspectors and auditors. Organizations themselves use methods of control to ensure staff do what is needed to achieve organizational objectives, such as writing policies and having internal rules, and groups of employees instil behavioural expectations in each other through social norms and culture.

Accountability in both public and private organizations, therefore, has to encompass not only strategic decision making by the organization but also the values and the controls that the organization is expected to abide by. Poor results in terms of organizational success are not tolerated by society but neither are good results produced in unacceptable ways. The essence of accountability is, therefore, provided through the ability of the organization to demonstrate the moral and social integrity of its actions. When organizations or individuals are trusted, there tend to be few demands to demonstrate integrity. But if trust is low, organizations and individuals tend to be called to account – to demonstrate publicly that they are behaving in socially acceptable ways and delivering what is expected of them.

There are four different modes of control. Behaviour control, which is essentially control of processes, focuses on the process that turns appropriate behaviour into desirable outputs. In this, very simple, routine jobs are designed so that behaviours can be easily observed, and reward can be based upon the delivery of the right behaviours. In a management context, behaviour-based control is accomplished through job design (Eisenhardt 1985). The second form of control is output control, in which more complex, interesting jobs are designed. The organization can invest in information systems, e.g. budgeting systems or layers of management, in order to gain knowledge about behaviours and reward is based upon these behaviours (Eisenhardt 1985). This strategy can encourage the generation of a huge quantity of measures of performance and tends to be that most favoured by central governments. Output-based control requires close monitoring of performance and requires precise measures.

A third form, outcome-based control, requires the design of more complex, interesting jobs, but seeks a simpler evaluation scheme, e.g. profitability or revenues, and reward is based upon the results. The rewards are much riskier but there is less need for precise job design. This is more in line with professional service models, such as those of employing clinical professionals. With outcome-based control the employee bears more risk on behalf of the organization and, therefore, has more power within the organisation, being in a stronger bargaining position. It is intended to be motivational and is useful when behaviours are difficult to observe, although it does require a degree of risk sharing.

The fourth option is social or clan control, which requires employing people whose preferences coincide with those of management. This option emphasizes people policies such as selection, training and socialization in which members are committed to organizations and views are shared. It is particularly attractive when any kind of measurement is costly. However, its disadvantage is lengthy implementation time (Eisenhardt 1985). Generally, in health care, clan controls are very strong through professional socialization. However, in the past these have been found to be counterproductive to organizational management, in that the common values are not those of the organization but those of the professional group and frequently organizational and professional values conflict. The task of restructuring in the NHS in the past has been an attempt to remove professional clan control and replace it with organizational clan control.

Assurance by using controls starts from the recognition that people use mechanisms to control their behaviour in every aspect of their life but are not aware of them. When you left home today, did you lock your door? Do you balance your bank statement? Do you review your monthly credit card statement? Do you count the change given to you by shop assistants? These are but a few examples of things that people do in order to reasonably assure that the desired results (protected home, accurate bank and credit card balances, and correct change) are achieved. These checks can either be left to the individual to determine, or can be written out in checklists to be reviewed and ticked off. In either case, in theory, an external review of the processes of checking could be carried out, which would provide assurance to others that such controls were in place and being effective.

Like people conducting the business of their day-to-day affairs, organizations have similar concerns in the conduct of their daily business. Organizations, therefore, have to have systems, that is controls, in place to make sure that activities are carried out appropriately and to restrict actions that may present risks, that is actions which may directly or indirectly lead to harm or failure to achieve what the organization has set out to deliver (Das and Teng 2001). There are essentially two different approaches to organizational control – externally-imposed control and internally-generated control. Both external and internal controls can be sub-divided into two categories. The first is formal, that is measure-based control (such as the tick list) and the second, informal or value-based control, which requires conformity to expected behaviours (Eisenhardt 1985). The first approach, also called objective control, emphasizes the establishment and use of formal rules, procedures and policies to monitor and reward desirable performance. The second approach relies on 'the establishment of organisational norms, values, culture, and the internalisation of goals to encourage desirable behaviour and outcome. Here control is intended to reduce goal incongruence and preference divergence among organisational members. The second approach when used in relation to organisations rather than professional or social groups has been called informal control or normative control' (Das and Teng 2001 page 6). This is the softer end of management practice, ensuring that the values subscribed to by the organization are instilled in the people who work for it.

Formal and informal controls, therefore, can originate both inside or outside an organization. Some controls created externally, such as legislation and regulation, are imposed by governments or their agents to protect society or individuals. But it must be noted that the legislation and regulation exists simply to control human behaviour. Take, for example, the laws governing strategies for pest control where it is easy enough to pass laws, but this begs the question, how do you train the insects to obey them? In reality, of course, legal sanctions are aimed, not at the insects themselves, but at a range of human behaviours that are most likely to affect the dynamics of pest populations. Legal controls, therefore, include all forms of legislation and regulation that might encourage individuals to act in such ways as to reduce spread of an insect population. Other formal controls are created by monitoring or review bodies specifying what is required as good practice. Externally-generated controls tend to focus on formal controls as these tend to use high levels of prescription but it is also possible for external controls to be generated informally by clan culture, such as seen in health care by the dominance of expected conformity with professional value systems and professional behaviours, monitored by professional bodies such as the Royal Colleges.

Internal controls can also be both formal and informal. Requirements can be specified and turned into checklists following a formal control model. However, organizational culture is a powerful force, and can over-ride formal control systems. Organizational research has demonstrated how power and politics, the bedrock of organizational culture, can have a significant impact on the behaviour of individuals in organizations (Walsh and Schneider 2002). Therefore, any assessment of internal control has to encompass not only rules and regulations denoting appropriate or acceptable behaviour but also must recognize the psychological and human elements of behaviour. Internal controls must encompass the processes that organizations develop themselves to meet the requirements placed upon the organization for good and ethical behaviour (Walsh and Schneider 2002). Internal control is, therefore, the total management system that brings together as a coherent whole all the pressures put upon the staff of an organization to act in particular ways. All the actions of staff impact upon the ability of the organization to meet its objectives. A weak link at any level of the organization compromises the integrity of the internal control system Thus, the collective effort made toward the achievement of organizational objectives is referred to as the internal control system. The desire for the creation of a method that allows a systematic appraisal of the whole system of internal control, encompassing both the formally-specified processes and procedures and the informally-generated norms of behaviour, has been the driving force behind the development of recent approaches to audit.

The efficient and effective development and use of controls, formal and informal, leads to good governance and ensures risks are mitigated and businesses and organizations can demonstrate that they are acting responsibly to achieve their publicly-stated objectives. Corporate governance is, therefore, essentially about finding the best methods of control to deliver organizational goals (Das and Teng 2001). In complex organizations, where the senior management or member of the board cannot possibly know every detail of what is going on in their organization, systems must be created that control the activities of the people who work in them, and the board, to fulfil its role, must be responsible for the functioning of those systems. Therefore, for the board to be held to account, the board must be open to external scrutiny not only in its strategic decision making and its performance but also in the internal systems for which it is responsible.

Yet, systems work continuously and scrutiny of outputs and internal systems cannot be continuous. Therefore, there is a need for assurance, that is the process by which accountability is supported, in order to fill the vacuum where there is a lack of information about actions and processes from the times between audits. Through assurance received by the board that the organization is doing its 'reasonable best' to achieve its objectives in the right way, the board is able to provide an assurance to external stakeholders, including the public, about its direction and control of the organization. But how should the board of a health care organization provide such assurance, particularly when decision making is no longer prescribed by the centre? How can it demonstrate that it is striving to achieve the requirements placed upon it for good quality health care?

Assurance is a concept based upon a belief that an organization can account for its internal management processes. The concept of assurance has its origins in audit, which expects that an organization will present itself for external scrutiny. There are only two basic approaches to providing assurance. The organization can either open up its whole working to external review, such as that found in inspection, or it can conduct its own inspection of its internal workings and invite external assessment of its own inspection processes. In addition, the organization can either follow externally-imposed rules, such as those found in external regulation, or it can be left to its own devices to create its own internal rules for ensuring good practices and behaviours within the organization. These 'rules' define the organizational structures, processes and actions that cause the organization to deliver its objectives and these, therefore, constitute good management, and are frequently referred to as controls. It is these controls that form the basis for the production of assurance.

The language and concepts of organizational control are borrowed from engineering and from information processing, and are modified by management concepts and language. Frequently, management control systems are described as though they are engineering tools, and can be treated as such. However, management theory introduces the notion that organizational systems are created and run by the interactions of individual people and, therefore, it is necessary to remember that management difficulties always arise when individuals feel coerced into performing actions. Understanding organizational control, therefore, requires that the language of those who describe the systems and the motivations of those who seek to introduce them must be carefully examined and the reality distilled from the theory and the aspiration.

Risk and risk management

Control, therefore, exists to mitigate risk. Risk is most commonly held to mean 'hazard' and something to be avoided (Performance and Innovation Unit 2002). Risk management covers all the processes involved in identifying, assessing and judging risks, assigning ownership, taking actions to mitigate or anticipate risk; and monitoring and reviewing progress (National Audit Office 2000). Good risk management helps reduce hazard, and builds confidence to innovate. It is 'a systematic approach to setting the best course of action under uncertainty by identifying, assessing, understanding, acting on and communicating risk issues' (Treasury Board of Canada 2000 page 5).

Risk is frequently used to describe a situation in which randomness can be expressed in terms of specific numerical probabilities, which can either be expressed objectively or reflect individual subjective belief. In policy making and management, risk is more likely to be used simply to describe uncertainty of outcomes, and more specifically, when attempts are made to create approximate measures of risk, to allow different types of risk that may impact on the organization's objectives, to be compared. 'Risk refers to the uncertainty that surrounds future events and outcomes. It is the expression of the likelihood and impact of an event with the potential to influence the achievement of an organization's objectives' (Treasury Board of Canada 2000 page 4). The phrase 'the expression of the likelihood and impact of an event' implies that a quantitative or qualitative analysis is required for making decisions concerning major risks or threats to the achievement of an organization's objectives. For each risk, two calculations are required: its likelihood or probability; and the extent of the impact or consequences.

For businesses there has been a preference to define risk in strategic terms, as 'the possibility that an event will occur and adversely affect the achievement of objectives' (Chapman 2003 page 3, taken from the CoSo model of enterprise risk management). Risk management in organizations, therefore, tended to concentrate on making decisions that contributed to the achievement of an organization's objectives by applying it both at the individual activity level and in functional areas. Risk management in public services assists with decisions such as the reconciliation of science-based evidence and other factors and, more significantly, helps to make appropriate decisions in investing limited public resources in desirable outcomes.

Two types of uncertainty in handling risk have been identified: uncertainty as a result of a lack of information and uncertainty in terms of unpredictable events (Performance and Innovation Unit 2001b para 19). Definitions of risk in the management and policy context differ in how they characterize outcomes. Some describe risk as having only adverse consequences, while others are neutral (Treasury Board of Canada 2000). However, the Treasury and associated government departments have been keen to view risk as also including opportunity (HM Treasury 2000b page 2).

> Improving public services requires innovation – seizing new opportunities and managing the risks involved. In this context risk is defined as uncertainty of outcome, whether positive opportunity or negative threat, of actions and events. It is the combination of likelihood and impact, including perceived importance.
>
> (Cabinet Office 2002 page 7)

Today it is recognized that public service organizations face many different types of risk across the whole spectrum of management activity including policies, programmes, operations, projects, finances, human resources, technology, health, safety, national and local politics, and organizational reputation. Risks can also present themselves on a number of fronts ranging from high-level, high-impact risks to low-level, minor impact risks. All demand a co-ordinated, systematic corporate response, which requires an integrated risk management approach. It is no longer sufficient to manage risk at the level of individual activity, such as health and safety, or viewing risk as contained within functional silos.

> Integrated risk management is a continuous, proactive and systematic process to understand, manage and communicate risk from an organization-wide perspective. It is about making strategic decisions that contribute to the achievement of an organization's overall corporate objectives.
>
> (Treasury Board of Canada 2000 page 5)

Integrated risk management, sometimes called enterprise risk management or organization-wide risk management, requires an ongoing assessment of potential risks within an organization at every level and then aggregating the results at the corporate level to facilitate priority setting and improved decision making. Integrated risk management, it is argued, should become embedded in the organization's corporate strategy and shape the organization's risk management culture. The identification, assessment and management of risk across an organization helps reveal the importance of addressing the organization as an integrated whole: the sum of the risks and the interdependence of the parts. And risk management aims to achieve the optimal balance between activities that foster innovation, so that the returns on investment can be maximized in ways that minimize the risk of harm (Treasury Board of Canada 2000).

Governance and control structures are needed to ensure that the organization has clearly-stated objectives, support in due diligence, is responsible in its risk-taking and innovation and, therefore, can deliver accountability by demonstrating that the board and its management and staff are able to handle risks effectively and appropriately. As noted earlier, assurance to underpin accountability is predicated on the assumption that a board or an organization has done its 'reasonable best' to meet its objectives. The concept of 'reasonable best' is crucial to the understanding of assurance. It depends upon the board being able to demonstrate it has assessed a risk and determined the most effective and appropriate action to deal with the risk. In this case, the costs of action must be weighed against the assessment of the severity and the likelihood of the risk.

> Investing in ever-greater rail safety measures beyond what is reasonably practicable under the Health and Safety at Work Act, for example, would be likely to put up rail fares, and have implications for both access charges paid by train operators and Government subsidy. It could also lead to greater use of the roads. This would in turn lead to more transport-related deaths.
>
> (Better regulation task force 2003 page 20)

However, the current approach to accountability used by government departments, combined with their inability to manage risk successfully, has been considered to be undermining innovation and change and, therefore, not able to deliver the expected outcomes required of modern public services.

> Accountability mechanisms are perceived by some in government as a discouragement to innovate and change, but this appears to be only one of a number of complex factors, including a lack of incentives to

manage risks, and a lack of commercial decision making skills within departments.

(Lord Sharman 2002 Para 5.35)

Trust

The concept of trust, with regard to the public's relationship to the actions of government, is regarded with growing concern – although there is little clarity as to what it means. In this context, however, it conveys a subjective judgement concerning the confidence of an individual in another person, or indeed an institution or organization. It is not necessarily based upon knowledge or factual information but upon faith that actions will be conducted with one's best interests in mind. Trust is an important component of accountability. If trust is undoubted, there will be no questions asked about the motivations or the actions of others or organizations. Where trust is more circumspect, an individual or organization is held to account by being asked to explain their actions, and even then there must be trust in their truthfulness. If trust is lacking, there will be a greater need for information to verify the claims of the individual or the organization about their actions.

Trust has become increasingly important given the emphasis upon modernization and the need for change. 'In a world of increasing uncertainty and complexity, flat hierarchies, more participative management styles and increasing professionalism, trust is thought of to be a more appropriate mechanism for controlling organisational life' (Sydow 1998 page 31). Trust, therefore, is associated with autonomy, which is deemed to equate with responsible actions. Trust in public bodies is also associated with the quality of services experienced by individuals, and how open and honest organizations are and how willing they are to learn from their mistakes (Audit Commission 2003 page 8). For organizations, however, there has to be what is termed systemic trust, based on structures and intra- and inter-organisational relationships, which provide predictability in their actions and outcomes; rather than personal trust, based upon familiarity between individuals (Garsten and Grey 2001). Public trust in public institutions, therefore, derives from the appropriate provision of accountability, which enables central government and public services to demonstrate how they are making decisions and delivering policies and services.

There is an inexorable progression of logic in these arguments. In order to improve public trust in organizations and individuals, it is necessary for them to be able to be held to account – to demonstrate they are capable of public trust. Accountability requires the ability to show not only good outcomes but also acceptable means of achieving the outcomes. The Nolan report, which set out the principles of public life, described the values associated with honourable and trustworthy behaviour: (un)selfishness, integrity, objectivity, accountability, openness, honesty and leadership (Lord Nolan and his committee 1995). Acceptable means require not only adherence to legal requirements and social values but also encompasses the expectation that organizations and individuals will not put themselves, other interested parties, or society at large at risk of harm. And risk of harm covers a range of possibilities, ranging from physical harm or hazard, to inappropriate stewardship of public resources, to damaging social stability and public confidence and failure to deliver the political agenda of the day.

Trust, however, is a multilevel phenomenon (Das and Teng 2001 page 4) because it is found in personal, organizational and inter-organizational relationships. Although there are some views that trust is based in knowledge and certainty (that is in the predictability of certainty in actions and outcomes and, therefore, based on performance according to agreements), for the most part, discussions of trust are based on perceptions of a willingness to act in certain way, known as 'good will'. Risk is held to play an important role in the understanding of trust: 'Without uncertainty in the outcome, trust has no role of any consequence' (Das and Teng 2001 page 6). Good will, therefore, is about good faith, good intentions and integrity: 'Good will trust delineates only a firm's intention to make things work, rather than one's ability to accomplish that' (Das and Teng 2001 page 6). Therefore, accountability, when considered in relation to trust, must require that an organization can demonstrate that it is doing its best to be worthy of trust – that is, its intentions and its processes are good. Mistakes do happen and errors do occur. Therefore, it is necessary to promote good will trust. However, poor performance, sustained over a long period of time, will erode good will trust.

This leads to the models of accountability that are contained in current audit thinking. Accountability can best be delivered through an examination of governance processes. But, sometimes, things can go wrong and it is not fair necessarily to judge the governance of organizations solely on outcomes. Some outcomes are so unpredictable or driven by external events that they could not have been foreseen or managed. Recent ideas of corporate governance are based upon the idea that the organization should be judged on its ability to manage, given the risks it has identified. The organization is only justified in failing to manage appropriately if it can demonstrate that it either, reasonably did not foresee the risks, or it had identified the risk but had put in place a reasonable, but in the event, insufficient approach to managing the risk.

Therefore, if management responsibility for running health care is to be devolved away from central government, it is necessary to question which approach to control is appropriate to deliver public accountability. This requires an understanding of appropriate control and how it is to be used both to deliver the health care required by the general public and to provide the necessary assurances for accountability. In the past, the NHS has relied upon the various different forms of control that have arisen expediently – behavioural control through job design, output control through central government assessment of performance, and clan control through the workings of its different professional organizations. These have facilitated the management of the health service but they no longer are trusted to provide the form of assurance necessary to replace public trust and to deliver the new requirements of accountability. A new approach to understanding control in health care is required.

Examining controls

The options for assurance-based control can be classified into four main types: formal or objective, external control; informal or value-based, external control; formal or objective, internal control; and informal, values-based internal control (see Table 2.2). These four types of control are aimed at ensuring that the behaviour of individuals, normally within an organizational setting, conform to expected definitions of what is safe, ethical and socially acceptable. These types of control are rarely used in isolation. Rather, combinations of the different types exist, creating the appropriate balance of specification of control and its assessment. The key issue is the creation of an appropriate mixture of formal and informal control, which does not over-burden organizations with administration but which permits the appropriate level of assurance to be created.

External control

The most dirigiste form of control imposed externally is that of legislation and regulations or rules, which exist in order to control the activities of individuals

Table 2.2 Types of control

	External control	*Internal control*
Formal control	Legislation and centrally-imposed regulation – national control on the management of risks	Organizational control on the management of risks
Informal control	Professional value systems – national clan controls	Organizational culture – values-based controls

and organizations, both private and public sector. This is sometimes referred to as formal or objective control. Regulation may be defined as any government measure or intervention that seeks to change the behaviour of individuals or groups by promoting the rights and liberties of citizens and restricting what they can do (National Audit Office 2001b). Formal control can include the specification of organizational structures and processes when these are included in standards used for the inspection of organizations.

External control can also be imposed in a less formalized way through the imposition of group values upon groups working within organizations. This is external control imposed by bodies or organizations other than government, who seek to impose clan norms on the behaviour of individuals (such as that exercised by professional bodies, peer review organisations, etc.) and includes those behaviours required by individual professionals to discharge their professional responsibilities. This is referred to as values-based external control and is frequently based upon processes of self-regulation and professional controls on training, and the development of norms and values within the members of the profession or group. This can also include the specification of standards used for the review of organizational or individual professional activity.

Internal control

These are processes prescribed for management to follow in order to achieve audit and other external assessment requirements. They are prescriptions covering, for example, good practice requirements. This includes the creation of policies and procedures by the management of organizations, which may be used to ensure legislation is met or organizational policies are followed and is, therefore, a form of formal or objective control applied internally within organizations. Internal control in this form is the province of internal auditors who are employed purely to examine internal control processes. Managers and auditors alike are exhorted to identify adequate control, which in turn is defined in terms of the plans and organizational structures that provide reasonable assurance that organizational objectives will be achieved effectively and economically. The aim is to ensure that control is effective, that is it is management-directed, authorized and monitors performance, which includes comparing actual with planned performance on a regular basis, and documenting these actions to provide reasonable assurance that organizational goals will be achieved. Any review system should provide what is termed 'reasonable assurance' to the public and other stakeholders that the internal control systems are working correctly. In other words, assurance, that errors and other deviations are kept to a tolerable level; for example, in the normal course of their assigned duties, employees will prevent errors or improper acts or will detect and correct them within a reasonable time, thereby mitigating their detrimental effects.

Whereas formal controls specify precisely what is required of organizations to demonstrate systems and processes, social groups create informal, internal controls. These are the product of people working together and creating social norms and values that influence, and in fact, control what they do. Because individuals at any level of the organization can affect the workings of internal controls, informal processes used to control individual behaviour become important. It is argued that the stronger the informal internal controls, the less prescription is needed for formal control systems. Indeed, management theory favours encouraging people to adopt behaviours willingly through internalizing values and norms of behaviour, rather than having to operate to written rules and procedures. This is particularly important in the team-based, professional activities required to deliver health care. According to Ouchi (1979), social control is most appropriate in high trust situations and also advances trust. But trust between the public services and the general public is now fragile and for accountability to be advanced, the case has been made for an improved system of assurance (Ouchi 1979). Boards have to determine the appropriate balance of trust and monitoring required for these new public services and how it is best achieved (Das and Teng 2001).

Values-based, internal control is, therefore, the culture that exists within an organization, which determines how the individuals working within the organization function, how they interpret and adhere to rules and procedures, how they inculcate values for ethical behaviour and treating each other properly. The internalization of good behaviour is the product of good leadership. Informal internal control is in line with management thinking, which seeks to bring out the best in the people who work within systems. It is argued that there are alternatives to reliance on external controls, pushing and threats – implied or real. If people are committed to shared values, they will exercise self-direction and self-control in the service of the organization's objectives.

Assurance of control types

Control may originate inside or outside the organization but the responsibility for demonstrating that the organization is conducting itself appropriately can also be placed inside or outside the organization (see table 2.3). Therefore, demonstrating compliance with legislation or externally-imposed regulations can either be conducted by external inspection bodies or left to the organization to produce its own assessment of how well it complies. This assessment process can be verified by independent assessors, such as auditors or inspectors. It is, therefore, necessary to consider the appropriate combination of assurance against controls. External control can use external review processes, such as inspection and audit, to provide assurance. Here, assurance can be

Table 2.3 Types of assurance

Assurance processes	External control	Internal control
External assurance	Inspection using standards or judgement	Internal audit using checklists for the structure of internal control
Internal assurance	Internal review using standards or judgement	Internal audit using self-assessment workshops

based either on the judgements of experts in a particular field, who understand the issues and the nuances of service delivery and professional expertise that tend to dominate health services. However, this form of review requires professional resources which could be better used providing services and also, given the dependence upon the judgement of individuals, is difficult to demonstrate consistency in judgement using this method. As a major concern in accountability in health care is the demonstration of equity in treatment, consistency is considered to be very important. In addition, systematic review is also held to be an important component of accountability, in which it can be demonstrated that the same inspection procedure is applied routinely and precisely to all organizations and circumstances.

Inspection can be based upon organizational standards and checklists that provide detailed specifications of what is required by organizations in terms of structures and policies. 'The indicators of quality tend to be features of the physical and organisational structure of the institution and the criteria/ standards are formulated accordingly' (Donabedian 1986). Or inspection could use detailed checklists, not to prescribe the structures and processes of organizational and service delivery systems but to describe the internal monitoring systems for the organization. This is, in effect, quality assurance of quality control and can be focused on either internal quality assurance processes or, indeed, internal quality improvement processes. External specification of systems, whether service delivery or quality assurance, enable greater consistency in the review process but tend to be highly prescriptive and restrict organizational development and innovation because they require conformity to detailed specifications. This runs counter to the arguments in the modernization agenda for greater freedoms to find solutions at the local level. An alternative is to permit organizations to check their own actions against externally-agreed checklists and to then submit their assessment processes for external scrutiny, using auditors or inspectors trained to recognize the components of good systems. Again, this raises questions about the difficulty of maintaining consistency across individual inspectors or auditors. It is, therefore, necessary to find the appropriate balance between the specification of quality and its assessment, in order to produce acceptable accountability.

Which approach to follow?

In the new policy environment of devolved management – of standards and standardization – which of these approaches is the best to follow? Which will generate the best form of assurance that is compatible with the vision of improved health care, capable of modernization in terms of meeting increasing public expectations for better quality and more choice, free from central control but still able to be held democratically accountable?

Management theory has long argued that individuals should be encouraged to choose to deliver their best, rather than be coerced through rules. In recent times, ideas about controls in management have become less restrictive, reflecting both greater individualism in choice and suggesting the need to guide individuals into managing appropriate choices in behaviours that carry risks (Walsh and Schneider 2002). Therefore, there has to be a change in the way the three main parties in the delivery of public services – the government, the service providers and the public – relate to each other. The government has to be willing to let go of central control to promote a greater degree of interaction between the public and the service providers. The public has to adapt its expectations to recognize that service providers do their best but may make mistakes. There has to be an agreement about what are acceptable circumstances in which mistakes may be made: that is, where risks may occur and not be able to be controlled. In addition, the service providing organizations have to ensure their staff understand the values of customer service within the culture of the organisation by committing to clear organizational values.

The emphasis on organizational and corporate culture, popularized by Peters and Waterman (1982), is thought to have been a direct product of a desire to reduce bureaucracy, substituting organizational values for rules. In this way, values have been recognized as an alternative form of control, achieved through enrolling individuals into corporate values and committing them to a set of universally-agreed corporate objectives (Garsten and Grey 2001). In turn, the government has to recognize corporate and consumer values as the main controls upon the delivery of quality services and develop a new relationship with both companies and public sector organizations. Tony Blair, in his famous speech on stake-holding (referred to as the Singapore speech, in reference to where he gave it), emphasized the new developments in governance, suggesting that there had to be what he called the right relationship of trust between businesses or public sector organizations and government. The government has to move from a position of dirigiste control to enabling organizations to develop the best relationships with their consumers.

For far too long, relations have been dogged by the fear that business left to its own devices will not be socially responsible. In reality, in a modern economy, we need neither old style dirigisme, nor rampant laissez faire. There are key objectives on which business and Government can agree and work together to achieve. This 'enabling' role of Government is crucial to long term stability and growth.

(Blair 1996)

Governments therefore, have had to rethink how they develop an appropriate relationship with service organizations, to ensure they provide what the public wants both in terms of service quality and accountability to implement the modernization agenda. To achieve this requires a change in the view of corporate governance. To do this, they have had to seek ways to empower public services, including health services, to facilitate the development of trust within the local public in both the decision making of government and the public services. Members of the public are much more aware of environmental and societal hazards and how these affect them. Public expectations for service delivery have increased and there are greater demands for involving the public in making decisions about the provision of public services.

Any government or regulatory body that seeks to control the behaviour of organizations confronts three basic choices. First, should controls be imposed centrally, creating standardization of acceptable behaviour or should they be allowed to develop locally (that is within the organization or a cluster of organizations), allowing cultural elements characteristic of individual communities to develop and control behaviour? There are arguments in favour of both, and typically a compromise between the two is sought. The second choice is the extent of specification that is required in determining controls. Should controls be highly specified, laying down policies and procedures to be followed in all circumstances or should there a 'lighter touch', trusting people and organizations to follow agreed principles but interpret them to enable them to meet their own particular objectives. Again, there are arguments in favour of both approaches. Over-specification prevents people and organizations from being free to innovate and find better solutions to service delivery and production processes. But too little specification creates the opportunity for unsafe and unacceptable practices to become cultural norms. The key issue here is finding the appropriate balance between specification of behaviours and freedom. The third choice concerns the provision of assurance. How can appropriate and acceptable behaviours be demonstrated to exist? How can an organization or an individual demonstrate that, not only have they managed to escape being caught breaking the law or acting in an unacceptable manner, but also that they have positively pursued good behaviour and are, therefore, acting in a socially appropriate manner. As later chapters will demonstrate, although this is a concern for private sector organisations, it is much more of a concern for public sector organizations, particularly those involved in health care. These organizations are perceived to operate under a duty to demonstrate that they are continuously striving to meet public expectations and to be safe, relevant and appropriate for the populations they serve.

Governments have also had to recognize the lack of precision encountered in the definition of risks and their impact, which arises from the increasingly complex societal issues that policy making and the management of public services must address. Governments are concerned with the protection of citizens from a wide variety of risks including: direct threats, such as the threat of chemical and biological attack, or accident, or the breakdown of information technology systems; safety issues, such as BSE, the MMR vaccine, flooding, or rail safety; risks to the environment from climate change or pollution; risks to the delivery of 'a challenging public service agenda'; the transfer of risk in capital projects and service delivery to and from the private sector; 'ambitions to make the public sector more innovative and better able to judge risks that might deliver high rewards'; the risk to the government's reputation in the eyes of the public (Cabinet Office 2002).

These issues directly impact upon the making of policy and the management of health care. Governments are seeking ways of improving the handling of the public in dealing with risks to society through better consultation and regulatory decision making; the improved operational management of public services to ensure safer delivery of services; and improved public management from within the civil service, as well as in health care management, through better strategic planning and performance management, which recognizes the centrality of patients in the delivery of health care. In short, there is a search for improved methods of control, and understanding of the role of controls, in the delivery of services including health services.

However, it is also necessary to consider the extent to which information is made available to the public or to interested parties in the achievement of accountability. To what extent is it enough to know that inspection or review has taken place and been found adequate, or to what extent should the findings be made public to allow the public and others to judge the adequacy of the system? The role of the auditor is to make a judgement about whether the organization has done what it set out to do. The role of a regulator is to act as both jury and judge, in that the regulator can not only determine whether compliance has occurred but also determine the sanctions to be applied. The role of an inspector is, in theory, more neutral, in that this role merely provides information or failure to comply, which is then acted upon by the appropriate bodies located within the accountability system (a process that exists in the formal structures of the public sector).

> We see accountability as a relationship based on the provision of information about performance from those who have it to those who

have a right to it, either because they have the power to reward or sanction, or because they have a 'right to know'. As a formal device, it includes both agent responsibilities (to inform) and principal responsibilities (to incentivise – to reward or sanction). Its primary responsibility is to close the performance loop.

(Anderson and Dovey 2003 page 5)

The previous chapter discussed the complex nature of service quality. Service quality as a concept is based upon the extent to which the experience of services meets with personal expectations of service. Where services fail to come up to expectations, the perception of service quality is eroded. Word of mouth comments on poor service quality will damage the image and reputation of the organization. Similarly, this chapter has demonstrated that trust is based upon expectations that an organization will attempt to deliver quality services and to make decisions appropriately, at all levels of the organization. When organizational performance is demonstrated through media reporting of incidents and adverse events or repeated comments on poor quality, public trust in the organization is similarly eroded. To maintain trust the organization must be able to demonstrate that its processes are designed to deliver good quality and good performance, and when things go wrong must be able to explain that errors were due to unforeseen circumstances. Accountability in terms of honest reporting of performance is essential for public trust but it is also important for processes, that is controls, to be well managed, in order to sustain public trust when either performance is hard to measure or to explain, or when things go wrong.

Understanding and communicating about control is also vitally important to delivering choice in health care. Patients need to be able to choose not only the time and the type of health care but also the nature of the care and treatment they receive. They need to be assured that the health care systems in which they are placing their faith – and their health and well-being – are well managed and will deliver health care in the way that patients want and expect. Governments cannot control centrally all the actions of organizations for which they are responsible. They have to find an appropriate balance between central control and local and professional freedom to take action, which will enable both the delivery of health care in the form that is acceptable to the general public and the delivery of health care that ensures that the individual patient is placed at the centre of any decision about treatment. The following chapters will examine the experience of trying to develop control and provide assurances in the private sector, central government and in the National Health Service, to establish which is the preferred option for health care systems of the future.

The story of the development of ideas about control starts, in Chapter 3, in attempts to regulate the activities of businesses – the need to generate better methods of governance that provide for both public concerns about safety and doing well, and yet do not detract from the freedoms that must be accorded to private businesses or their equivalent to develop and grow and introduce improvements in the delivery of health care for the benefit of individual patients.

Chapter summary

This chapter has dealt with the following points:

- The inherent difficulties in reducing regulation while maintaining consistent quality of service.
- How accountability can be achieved through corporate governance.
- A discussion of different types of control, highlighting those methods used in controlling quality in health care systems.
- The impact of risk, risk management and trust on how the public perceives the quality of a health care service.
- The options for assurance-based control and which approach to follow.

---

3 The Emergence of Internal Control: Control in Private Businesses

Regulation, that is the application of formal external control through legislation (classic regulation) (Better regulation task force 2003 page 12), and regulations on the behaviour of private sector organizations have been in existence for centuries. But by the end of the 1990s, growing concerns were being expressed that government regulation of businesses had become excessive (Ayers and Braithwaite 1992). It has not been proven if this was the case. Some argued that Britain was one of the least regulated of all the affluent countries. Even so, regulation is a luxury that can only be afforded by prosperous populations.

> Only rich countries can afford the cost of anti-discriminatory and fair labour market regulations. Whereas regulation in the past was at the centre of an ideological debate between Marxism and liberal capitalism, today's debate takes place between the risk averse 'socially responsible' middle classes and the liberal capitalists. Ironically, although liberal capitalism appears to have prevailed over Marxism, it has had to moderate its own ideology in order to placate the readers of the Daily Mail.
>
> (Better regulation task force 2001 page 3)

Notwithstanding the disagreement about the extent of regulation in Britain compared with other countries, there was a popular and growing belief that so enthusiastic had been government departments at protecting the public interest that regulations were in danger of choking enterprise. 'Entrepreneurs were being distracted from running and growing their businesses by the cumulative burden of taxation, employment, public protection and environmental regulation' (Better regulation task force 2000b). These concerns were also extended to the public sector organizations that are regulated by government bodies: 'The way the Government regulates bodies within the public sector can also result in a disproportionate administrative burden' (National Audit Office 2001b Para 1.12). Not only was the burden of administrative regulation growing, there was also growing concern that it was not possible to enforce the regulations. It was increasingly recognized that it was difficult to provide assurance to politicians and taxpayers that organizations were complying with the extensive set of rules and regulations applied to them (National Audit Office 2001b). Government departments were facing a dilemma about protecting the health and safety of individuals or society, while at the same time appearing to be ineffective in enforcing their wishes.

At the Public Inquiry into the *Herald of Free Enterprise* disaster, Lord Justice Sheen was highly critical of the ferry operating company and found that 'from top to bottom the body corporate was infected with the disease of sloppiness' (Sheen 1987). Despite this finding, the prosecution for corporate manslaughter brought against the ferry company failed, leading to concerns about the inability to hold directors to account for accidents caused by the companies for which they are responsible (Culpin 2001). This case did establish the principle that a company could be guilty of manslaughter if it could be proved that an individual person, sufficiently senior in the company's hierarchy as to be part of the company's 'directing mind', had been guilty of serious negligence. However, since then there have been only three successful convictions for corporate manslaughter, even though there has been a significant number of high profile tragedies: Piper Alpha, Kings Cross London Underground Fire, Clapham Junction, Southall and Paddington rail crashes. The difficulty in pursuing prosecutions of directors has centred around the problems of identifying a single person as a 'controlling mind'. The growth in the number of accidents and safety failures led to pressure in the UK to increase director culpability in the control of hazards and risks, thereby making individual directors more responsible for, and more directly concerned with, the safety of the organization and the services and products it produces. Increasingly, legislation has been introduced to impose duties on companies and directors personally (ROSPA 2000).

Making board-level directors personally responsible and capable of prosecution is one solution but it places an onerous burden on individuals. An alternative and more popular approach within the private sector has been to identify board-level responsibilities in terms of the success of the board in running all aspects of its organization – what has now become known as corporate governance. A national report from South Africa on corporate governance, the King Report, advanced the opinion that 'corporate governance practices should reflect a committed effort to reduce workplace accidents, fatalities and occupational health and hygiene-related incidents' (The King Committee 2001 Page 116). Rather than recourse to legal sanctions, the King Report suggested there should be 'regular measurement against bare minimum legislative and regulatory requirements' (The King Committee 2001 page 116).

That is, to apply external review or inspection mechanisms to assess whether regulations are complied with.

Inspection, however, is an expensive activity and can open the gateway to over-specification of the practices required by organizations. Given that the private sector is made up of thousands of independent organizations, each required to ensure the minimization of a range of hazards, it became common to focus on the overall running of the governance of organizations. The governance role was considered not to be concerned with running the business of the company per se, but instead with giving overall direction to the business, with overseeing and controlling the executive actions of management and with 'satisfying legitimate expectations for accountability and regulation by interests beyond the corporate boundaries. If management is about running business, governance is about seeing that it is run properly. All companies need governing as well as managing' (Tricker 1984).

Corporate governance in different countries

The view that boards are able to determine whether their own management systems are satisfactory derives from an assumption about the role of the free market in ensuring acceptable behaviour by businesses. Competition between companies is the preferred mechanism to ensure companies deliver services and products that are needed in the market place (Gamble and Kelly 2001 page 113). If companies do not deliver what the market wants, the market will not purchase their products. Given the difficulty in defining quality, particularly in service businesses, regulations tended to focus only on the safety of individuals or society at large, leaving the experiential dimensions of quality to the producer to control and determine.

Shareholders own the company and, therefore, will ensure that the company behaves in such as way as to maximize their interests. Shareholders, therefore, expect the company to comply with laws and regulation and to understand and meet the needs of their consumers through good governance and good market performance, leaving the market to judge satisfaction with the product or service. An alternative model suggests instead that it is the duty of directors to maximize shareholder value because shareholders bear the residual risks of the enterprise. Therefore, only shareholders have the right to choose directors and to receive information that enables them to monitor their performance. The shareholder in both cases, by virtue of owning the company, will determine what is acceptable behaviour and will ensure that the company does whatever it needs to do to maximize consumer satisfaction (Easterbrook and Fischel 1996).

In the USA, corporate control is strongly influenced by the takeover market and discussions of governance are dominated by discussions of the impact of the separation of ownership and management (Franks and Mayer 1997; Monks and Minow 1994). It is assumed managers know what shareholders expect and shareholders can get enough information to judge whether their expectations are met. If not they would sell their shares. The separation of ownership from management could potentially lead to problems in ensuring that the agents of the shareholders, that is the management, act in the best interests of the shareholders. Corporate governance activities and structures, such as monitoring and control by non-executive directors and the design of suitable incentive mechanisms, have been introduced to keep management in check. The ultimate sanction that enables these mechanisms to be effective is the market for corporate control itself (Garrod 1996).

In many European countries, in contrast, corporate governance relies more heavily on monitoring of the actions of management by committee. The European tradition is to have two-tier boards, with a supervisory board where half of the members are elected by shareholders and the other half by the employees and labour unions, and a management board, which is appointed for a fixed term by the supervisory board. Considerable discretion is granted to management in day-to-day activities, and the supervisory board only intervenes when management is clearly shown to be unsuitable or unsuccessful (Garrod 1996).

In the UK and Canada there has been a further different emphasis. The concept of corporate governance in these countries has been dominated by issues regarding the shareholder-director relationship and the means to ensuring effective governance has been the structure of boards of directors and their sub-committees. In the UK, this resulted in calls for the professional self-regulation of a board of directors and for an increase in the number and influence of non-executive directors whose powers and responsibilities are not differentiated in the Companies Acts (1985 and 1989) from those of executive directors. Much greater emphasis is placed on professional self-regulation and private institutional shareholder-company communication than is the case in a market dominated by the takeover threat (Garrod 1996). In this model, the duty of the board is to 'supervise, direct or oversee', whereas day-to-day management must be delegated to others (Joint Committee on Corporate Governance 2001 page 12).

> The Board selects the CEO, and if it is to add value, it must work with senior management as collaborators in advancing the interests of the corporation. In doing so, it must delegate authority and recognize that, once authority is delegated, management must be free to manage. But the board cannot be too accepting of management's view. It has the responsibility to test and question management assertions,

to monitor progress, to evaluate management's performance and, where warranted to take corrective action.

(Joint Committee on Corporate Governance 2001 page 12)

The UK and Canadian models of corporate governance were based on a belief that better governance processes rather than structures, would promote better company performance. Sir Adrian Cadbury, in promoting the need for better governance in health care organizations, quotes from research evidence (Millstein and MacAvoy 1998), which claimed it proved the link between governance and performance (Cadbury 1993). Poor performers were found to have weak governance arrangements, which led to the assumption that better governance would lead to better performance (Cadbury and The London Stock Exchange 1992 Para 36). Therefore, businesses should be required to demonstrate they follow best practice in governance in order to maintain the confidence of their shareholders and the markets in which they operate.

However, this view is contested in research evidence (Heracleous 2001). Dr Jeanne Patterson shows that there were two important studies on boards in 1998 (by Millstein and MacAvoy) and in 1999 (by Bhagat and Black). Both studies looked at the active, independent board but the methodology and conclusions were different. Bhagat and Black studied 928 large US public companies in various subperiods from 1985 to 1995 and concluded that there was no convincing evidence that greater independence results in higher performance, but there was some evidence that firms with supermajority independent boards (with only one or two inside directors) performed worse than other firms. Millstein and MacAvoy, in their study of 154 large firms in 1995, concluded that there is a statistically significant relationship between active, independent boards and superior corporate performance (Millstein and MacAvoy 1998). Further research has failed to demonstrate a conclusive link between performance and governance but evidence has been produced to suggest that a more convincing argument is that while 'best practices' in corporate governance may be irrelevant to good performance, 'bad' practices may be more strongly related to underperformance; in other words, good governance may be a qualifier rather than a differentiator (Fama and Jensen 2000 page 168). This sort of evidence, plus the qualitative arguments in favour of the link between good governance and performance, brought wide spread support for the idea that good governance was an ideal to be pursued. However, the subject of corporate governance has become a concern probably not so much as the result of academic research but rather as the result of inquiries into the collapse of large corporations and the failure of chief executives throughout the 1980s (Tricker 1984).

Formalizing corporate governance

The need to formalize corporate governance, that is, the ways in which companies manage their internal operations, stemmed from concerns about the accountability of private firms due to increasing evidence that boards were ineffectual in the running of their companies and failing to take active responsibility for the strategic direction of their companies. In addition, although shareholders may be able to encourage the board of directors to deliver good performance, depending upon them to act to protect from harm employees, the public and society at large was, in general, not considered practical. Companies have wider public obligations that can be defined through the claims of different stakeholders in the company – including employees; suppliers; government; local, regional and national communities; banks; and shareholders. A form of self-regulation for companies to subscribe to was required, to assure their stakeholders that they were conducting themselves appropriately. As a result, 'Codes of best practice' were drawn up by several countries, global institutions and institutional investor organizations and adverse publicity created for companies with what were seen as ineffective governance systems – the premise for such action based on the fact that good governance means higher returns for share-holders and vice versa (Parkinson and Kelly 1999). These methods have been criticized for offering little more than an enlightened shareholder value perspective and, more importantly, for being a smokescreen for the continuation of unchecked managerial power. The London Stock Exchange, in its listing requirements, obliges companies to state how they applied the principles of a code of practice called the Combined Code. But the reality is that it is believed that while there should be accountability through having non-executive directors, the long-term health of the business is best secured if the primary responsibility is vested in the managers (Kay 1997).

Principles of sound financial corporate governance were being promulgated for the private sector in the UK and in other countries. In the UK, the first development was the Cadbury report, which recommended that the board of directors of each listed company registered in the UK should report on the effectiveness of the company's system of internal control (Cadbury and The London Stock Exchange 1992). In 1995, the Greenbury committee reported on the arrangements for paying directors and upheld the Cadbury principles of openness and transparency (Greenbury Committee 1995). In 1998, a successor committee to Cadbury recommended that an organization should not draw distinctions between internal financial control and other controls but should view the whole internal control system as a totality. The findings of these committees were consolidated into a single 'Combined Code of Principles of Good Governance', published by the London Stock Exchange

(London Stock Exchange 1998). In September 1999, the Internal Control Working Party of the Institute of Chartered Accountants, chaired by Nigel Turnbull, produced guidance on the internal control requirements of the Combined Code (Turnbull 1999). This report reinforced the principle that all controls, including risk management, should be the subject of review.

The private sector solution, therefore, has been to argue for methods to improve the internal control of the governance of organizations, that is, on the activities and the practices of boards in running their organisations, and to adopt voluntary codes to improve self-regulation by companies (Gamble and Kelly 2001 page 114). Essentially, this is a commitment to the concept of internal control, allowing companies to determine their own internal mechanisms for achieving compliance with legislation and seeking their own methods of providing assurance to their boards of good management practice, and using some form of verification of the assurance process by independent auditors. Using formal self-regulation, through Codes of Best Practice, to combat ineffective governance systems, based on the premise that good governance means higher returns for share-holders and vice versa (Parkinson and Kelly 1999). Adverse publicity would be created for companies with what are seen as ineffective governance systems, not only by shareholders but also wider stakeholders including: employees; suppliers; government; local, regional and national communities and banks. The Codes of Best Practice, if subject to audit scrutiny and external reporting, allow those interested in the running of the company to scrutinize its decisions.

Voluntary disclosure and external scrutiny are believed to be good mechanisms to check and change individual behaviour. Being observed can affect behaviour. 'Boards of directors are like subatomic particles – the behave differently when they are observed. And it never hurts to let them know they are being observed' (Minnow 2002). Not only does disclosure of performance and decision making provide examples of good practice that can be emulated by other organizations, but disclosure against guidelines can modify behaviour 'by forcing boards to focus explicitly on their roles and responsibilities and how they are being discharged' (Joint Committee on Corporate Governance 2001 page 10).

Good governance was, therefore, equated with board structure and conduct, but it was identified also as the ability of the board to manage the business properly. However, it was also necessary for the board to assure its various stakeholders, and the public at large, that it was in fact managing the business properly. The first major development in the provision of assurance was Steinberg's report (1993) of the Committee of Sponsoring Organisations (COSO) of the national commission on Fraudulent Financial Reporting (The Treadway Commission) which, in September 1992, identified that what was needed was 'a method for achieving rational assurance that objectives in areas related to the effectiveness and efficiency of operations, reliability of financial reports and compliance with laws and regulations are met'. The report labelled this 'internal control'. The report aimed to develop a system of organization-wide risk management that would enable a board to understand how to handle risk and the internal controls necessary to manage risk, and also how to explain to stakeholders what they were doing.

Internal control systems

As part of a standardized approach to the development of internal control systems, Steinberg's report identifies the five interrelated components of internal controls: the control environment; risk assessment; control activities; information and communication; and monitoring (Steinberg 1993). It suggests that these components are linked to the way in which management operates its business and are integral to the management process, and that they are linked not in a linear or serial fashion but as a multidirectional, interactive process. Each organization's internal control needs differ – depending upon the size, management philosophy, industry and culture of the business. Therefore, no two enterprises will have identical control systems. This conclusion is significant because it suggests that there cannot be a single approach to the specification of control systems.

Boards and their auditors are charged, therefore, with the task of determining whether a particular internal control system is effective, in order to provide the required assurances. The assessment of effectiveness is a subjective judgement arrived at by a subjective evaluation of whether the components of internal control are present and functioning effectively. The solution advocated by the COSO model was that a board was effective in managing its internal control systems if it could provide assurance against the three main areas of operations, financial reporting and compliance (into which all organizational operating objectives could be classified). Assurance could be provided if: the board could demonstrate that they understand the extent to which operational objectives are being met; published, financial statements are prepared reliably; and applicable laws and regulations are observed. Thus, if the board and the auditors can agree that the internal controls function effectively, then there is reasonable assurance that the organization is well managed. (Committee of Sponsoring Organisations, the Treadway Commission 1992 page 16; The Canadian Institute of Chartered Accountants 2003).

The Treadway report had a great impact upon the private sector and generated a succession of reports, which attempted to introduce the notion of control into various sectors. In 1998, growing concerns about the supervision of banking procedures led to the production of a general framework for the evaluation of internal control systems produced by the Basle Committee on Banking supervision. (Basle Committee on Banking Supervision 1998).

The Basle Committee is a committee of banking supervisory authorities, established by the central bank governors of the Group of Ten countries (Belgium, Canada, France, Germany, Italy, Japan, Luxembourg, Netherlands, Sweden, Switzerland, United Kingdom, and the United States) in 1975. The committee had been established to offer guidance on discussions of internal control systems in specific areas of banking, for example, interest rate risk or trading and derivatives activities (particularly pertinent after significant losses had been experienced by several banking organizations during the 1980s and 1990s). Analysis of the causes of the losses had caused banking supervisors to conclude that the losses could have been prevented, or at least detected much earlier (thus limiting the damage to the banks), had there been effective control systems. Although the committee recognized that each country should develop its own methods for monitoring internal control systems, using external auditors to also assess the systems, it was decided that there should be a number of general principles – 14 in total – by which a bank's internal control systems should be assessed.

In Canada, a similar initiative also created a model for the assessment of internal control known as: the Criteria of Control (CoCo), devised by the Board of the Canadian Institute of Chartered Accountants in 1995. This differed from its USA counterpart in a number of ways, mostly because it endeavoured to put control in a 'softer' or more human context (see table 3.1). Rather than creating a category of objectives for internal control, such as effectiveness and efficiency of operations, the Canadian model asks for an assessment of the effectiveness of the organization in achieving a specific objective, such as customer service. In addition, the Canadian model produced a series of 20 specific assessment criteria about how management and employees and others carry out their activities.

Table 3.1 CoCo criteria (Criteria of Control board of the Canadian Institute of Chartered Accountants 1995)

Purpose, i.e. the communication of the entity's objectives, the identification and assessment of the risks which may affect the objectives and the setting of policies and plans which should include measurable targets and indicators.

Commitment, i.e. shared ethical values, sympathetic human resource policies, defined authorities and responsibilities and an atmosphere of mutual trust.

Capability, i.e. knowledge and skill, communication processes and coordination of decision making.

Monitoring and learning, i.e. awareness of factors which could affect objectives now and in future, periodic challenge of current assumptions, monitoring performance against targets, initiating follow-up procedures where necessary and periodically assessing the effectiveness of internal control.

Significantly in the CoCo and the COSO approach to governance, internal control had become equated with the management of risks. It was argued that if an organization understood and managed the risks it faced while achieving its objectives, it would be in control.

However, it became apparent as the CoCo and COSO models were applied, that the subjective assessment of how well risks are managed and how well controls are embedded in organizations required a context for the assessment to be meaningful. Assurance needs to operate not only against the view of good internal control but also against a wider model of the objectives of the organization. People working in an organization need to know what they are supposed to be achieving. Similarly, a board has to have a clear view of why it exists and what it is there to achieve. 'If it cannot be clearly ascertained what is required from the company, it is impossible to determine when and whether specific goals have been met. Directors are concerned with the long term direction of their company. They need to set goals (or objectives) with varying time frames' (The Canadian Institute of Chartered Accountants 1995 para 19).

Setting and achieving objectives

The focus of concern for the development of internal control moved to identifying the objectives which were needed to provide the basis for the assurance framework. Mission statements and high-level goals are frequently produced as the rationale for companies but, it is argued, although valid these are too high level for actions to be judged against. 'Objectives . . . should be broken down into focused and achievable goals, against which is it easy to determine risks and to gauge when they have been met. For example, a specific objective might be to increase the customer base by 10% by way of superior customer service' (Centre for Business Performance 1999 page 8). Considerable advice has been offered in the control literature on how boards should approach the setting of objectives. It has been suggested that objectives should be future-oriented, that is, set in the future rather than the present. The board should ask itself whether the objectives it already has will meet the challenges that it is likely to face over at least the next two or three years (Centre for Business Performance 1999). When seen as part of strategic thinking, objective setting becomes a dynamic rather than a once-and-for-all activity.

> Objective setting involves identifying requirements that must be met, and identifying and balancing risks and opportunities associated with those requirements and the needs and wants of various parties (both internal and external). Objective setting thus requires an understanding of the organisation's mission and vision, the environment in which it operates and its position within that environment.

Objective setting is a continuous process, requiring monitoring of
operating performance and of changes in the internal and external
environments.

(The Canadian Institute of Chartered Accountants 1995 para 35)

This view of internal control provided a rationale for the existence of the
board of directors. If boards are to add value they must engage themselves
actively and regularly in the functions of strategic planning and risk management (Higgs 2003; Joint Committee on Corporate Governance 2001 page 21).
In addition, control is heavily dependent upon clear management structures
with evident lines of accountability for roles and responsibilities within
organizations.

Boards' involvement in strategic planning and the monitoring of risks
must recognize directors are not there to manage the business but are
responsible for overseeing management and holding it to account.
Where the lines are clear, and roles respected, effective boards will
contribute to the development of strategic direction and approve a
strategic plan. They will oversee the processes that management has
in place to identify business opportunities and risks. They will consider the extent and types of risk that it is acceptable for the company
to bear. They will monitor the management's systems and processes
for managing the broad range of business risk. And most important,
on an on-going basis they will review with management how the
strategic environment is changing, what key business risks and
opportunities are appearing, how they are being managed and what,
if any modifications in strategic direction should be adopted.

(Final report Joint Committee on Corporate Governance 2001
Page 21)

The role of the board is therefore clear – it is about overseeing management's strategic processes and making decisions on how the business should
be managed in the light of the risks it faces. Indeed, the current Toronto stock
exchange guidelines place even greater onus on the board of directors to identify the principal risks the organization is facing. The regulations state that the
board of directors for every corporation should explicitly assume responsibility for: a) adoption of the strategic planning process and b) the identification
of the principal risks of the corporation's business and ensuring the implementation of appropriate systems to manage these risks (Final report Joint
Committee on Corporate Governance 2001).

The objectives of an organization have an impact on more than the board
and the staff. Increasingly it is argued that the objective-setting process used
by businesses should be more inclusive of stakeholders, who have their own

interests and will wish to influence objectives. The board needs to balance the needs of the various interest groups, such as lenders, employees, customers and others, as well as the interests of shareholders and the meeting of regulatory requirements, and decide the best and most appropriate ways to address these (The Canadian Institute of Chartered Accountants 1995 para 36).

The focus of attention on ensuring the achievement of strategic objectives changed the way in which risk was thought of. Prior to this most management discussions of risk were concerned with unanticipated variation (i.e. downside risk) in business outcome variables, such as revenues, costs, profit market share and so forth (Miller 1992). However, the introduction of the idea of risk to strategic objectives required a broadening of the approach to risk away from just things that could go wrong, towards the failure to recognize and act upon opportunities for business development and growth, that is, to innovate and develop the business. 'Viewing risk from the opportunity perspective helps to highlight the inherent relationship between risk and return. The greater the risk, the greater the potential return and, conversely, the greater the potential for loss' (The King Committee 2001 page 100). Risk from an opportunity perspective is measurable in some circumstances, and qualitative in others. Strategic risk management, therefore, began to focus on how to deal with uncertainty – 'when considering issues from the perspective of uncertainty, companies should determine how they could prevent uncertain future events from having a negative impact. In other words, the management of uncertainty seeks to ensure that the company's actual performance falls within a defined range and is, of necessity, pro-active' (The King Committee 2001 page 100).

This approach to assessment of opportunities suggested that boards need to use more than just performance management to assess how effective their management is. It has been argued for a long time that managers tend to operate within 'bounded rationality' and, therefore, can only be expected to satisfice rather than optimize their outcomes (Simon 1991). They do not attempt to systematically review whether they are achieving the best outcomes and to review internal management systems in order to improve them. In addition, performance measures are designed to report past results rather than to predict future performance. By the time the performance measures have demonstrated a deterioration in results and the achievement of objectives, it is often too late to prevent losses or other adverse effects. (Centre for Business Performance 1999 page 18). Furthermore, most managers are not attuned to dealing with future performance and do not act on the basis of risk assessment. Managers have been thought to be insensitive to the estimates of probabilities of possible outcomes. Their decisions tend to be affected more by critical performance targets (March 1987). There was, therefore, an argument for reorienting management systems away from reviewing past performance to focusing on the future of the organization, which requires a shift in the attitude to risk management to a more optimistic, strategic planning approach. 'Risk management can be used to reinforce, on an ongoing basis, what senior management and the board are seeking to achieve. It is important that managers get out of an "only downside risk" mentality. Risk is not only "bad things happening" but also "good things not happening" ' (Centre for Business Performance 1999 page 6).

Risk and control

This change in thinking, in turn, forced a widening in the definition of internal control. Businesses have moved towards understanding that opportunities arise from focusing on risk and control, rather than purely focusing on controls (Centre for Business Performance 1999). It was recognized that control should cover the identification and mitigation of risks, and that these risks should not only include known risks related to the achievement of a specific objective. Thereby introducing two fundamental considerations that could impact on the viability and success of the organisation: these were 'a) failure to maintain the organisation's capacity to identify and exploit opportunities and b) failure to maintain the organisation's resilience. Resilience refers to the organisation's capacity to respond and adapt to unexpected risks and opportunities and to make decisions on the basis of telltale indications in the absence of definitive information' (The Canadian Institute of Chartered Accountants 1999 Annex A; Performance and Innovation Unit 2002).

However, companies and other organizations can have many different and frequently competing objectives and the elegance of a simple method of providing assurance on risk management across an organization was difficult to achieve. Some governance models hold the board responsible for all risks and specify that the board should be concerned with ensuring that internal control is integrated into all the activities of the company. 'Control should be established to encompass all possible management responses to risk. Controls are derived from the way management run the company and should be integrated into all business processes' (The King Committee 2001 page 100). The Turnbull report in the UK also focused upon the totality of an integrated, organization-wide control system, which covered the whole organization – from strategy, through operating systems, to protection of employees and customers from a wide range of risks (Centre for Business Performance 1999). Therefore a number of views evolved, which attempted to pull these various responsibilities into a single coherent system – otherwise known as enterprise risk management, or business risk management (Mackay and Sweeting 2000 page 368).

The approach adopted by the Turnbull Report expects that the review of the effectiveness of internal control, and the report to shareholders about it, should be from the perspective of the group as a whole. This led to the development of what has become known as organisation-wide or enterprise-wide risk management, in which risks would be managed throughout the organization and fed to the board. The key to enabling this system to work was the embedding of risk management and systems of internal control throughout the whole organization. Internal management systems would feed information on risks to the board, although indiscriminate generation and communication of risks could generate large numbers, which could, in turn, create an information overload for the board.

Focusing on too many risks could prevent the key, significant risks from receiving appropriate attention (Centre for Business Performance 1999). However boards are still responsible for risks of all kinds, including health and safety hazards within their organizations. Focusing solely on strategic risks, without ensuring compliance with safety regulations or observing financial probity requirements, could be equally damaging for companies. The board has to find mechanisms for distinguishing between risks that are perceived as significant at a local level but which will not have a major impact on the whole organization.

> Something significant to a local unit may not be significant to the organisation as a whole and something that seems insignificant to a local unit may however, be significant to the organisation as a whole. For example, one or two incidents of poor service to customers at a local unit level may take on significance to the organisation as a whole when considered in the context of the experiences of a number of local units or the potential of those customers to damage the reputation of the organisation.
>
> (Canadian Institute of Chartered Accountants 1997 para 44)

Therefore, customer complaints, for example, need to be reviewed carefully to establish whether a complaint is likely to highlight a problem that could undermine the business as a whole (Better regulation task force 2000a). There was a growing recognition that there was need to ensure that the board was alerted to all risks that might significantly affect the business (Centre for Business Performance 1999). But in addition, the risk management processes which deal with operational risks need to be joined with the strategic risk management process, to ensure a single, integrated risk management system. 'Care should also be taken to avoid two processes, one top down and one bottom up being performed independently of each other' (Centre for Business Performance 1999 page 9).

The alternative model was that companies should focus on selected, significant objectives and risk assessment should be directed to the organization's significant objectives. This should encompass significant business, strategic

and operational risks related to such objectives, including the failure to maintain resilience to respond to unexpected risks and the need to maintain
capacity to identify and exploit opportunities (The Canadian Institute of
Chartered Accountants 1995 page 5). However, boards could not be expected
to assess control for all conceivable objectives, or for all departments or units
(Canadian Institute of Chartered Accountants 1997).

It was also increasingly recognized that the introduction of organisation-
wide risk management, or enterprise risk management (ERM), was impossible
for most organizations. 'It's difficult, if not impossible, for most organisations
to expend the resources to develop their own enterprise risk management
process from scratch. In this day and age of lean and mean organisations, most
are struggling just to accomplish their day-to-day activities . . . They simply
don't have the time, talent, energy or money to undertake such a massive
project on their own' (Chapman 2003 page 2). As a consequence, the Committee of Sponsoring Organisations (COSO) of the Treadway Commission decided
to offer a single model for discussing and evaluating an organization's risk
management efforts. This was intended to incorporate, but not replace, the
integrated framework for internal control. This new risk management model
consists of eight components: internal environment; objective setting; event
identification; risk assessment; risk response; control activities; information
and communication; and monitoring. Five of the components overlap with
the COSO internal control framework, making the ERM 'a turbo-charged or
de-luxe version' of the internal control model (Chapman 2003 page 4).

The board is felt to have a duty to assess the conduct of the whole
organization – as well as ensuring that the individual functions for which it is
responsible are properly carried out by managers. This assessment, therefore,
does not duplicate or substitute the appropriate monitoring processes but it
does examine how the various elements within the organization are aligned:
'An assessment from the perspective of the whole is intended to assess but not
duplicate or substitute for, existing elements of control undertaken by an
organisation such as risk identification and assessment processes, strategic
planning and monitoring of external and internal environments' (Canadian
Institute of Chartered Accountants 1997 para 40). This, then, provided a
model in which boards could be free to manage their organizations to the best
of their ability, with freedom of management action, while ensuring appropriate levels of accountability to shareholders, stakeholders and other interested
parties. The board is required to identify that it has the right systems in place
(including adequate consultation) for planning and for identifying strategic
risks, which enable it to decide which objectives to pursue. But having identified these objectives, the board then needs to ensure that the organization is
capable of meeting them, and without putting itself (and the board) at risk of
failing to conduct itself properly. Therefore, the key to accountability is that
the board can ensure that the business is capable of identifying and managing

the specific risks that come from the operation of the business and which may cause it problems in the future. In addition, the board should have the right management features associated with good control systems to produce acceptable risk management. That is, not only are there good procedures in place throughout the organization but the culture of the organization, the quality of the staff and the quality of the leadership provided are considered good enough to deliver a company which is doing its best to succeed.

This is frequently described as the control environment – the context in which processes occur (Committee of Sponsoring Organisations – the Treadway Commission (COSO) 1992). It is not possible to assess processes independently of the environment in which they take place. The environment includes the attitudes, abilities, awareness and actions of the board and management regarding the significance of control within the organization, i.e. the 'tone at the top'. For example, poor training or a lack of adequate delegation of authority may negate the effectiveness of even the best control system. The control environment also includes the way in which information and communication systems provide management with reports detailing facts about operational, financial and compliance matters. The usefulness of information is determined by the attitude and the ability of staff to access it. Therefore, information must be relevant and communicated to appropriate personnel in a timely way for it to be useful, and information must flow in all directions within the organisation. The information and communication system helps to ensure that employees are aware of what is expected of them in accomplishing the organization's goals and objectives.

The view emerged that control could not be seen simply in terms of operational objectives, nor could it be easily contained within the COSO headings. Instead, there was a need to recognize the importance of culture in determining how well an organization can organize itself to achieve its goals. 'Effective control is as much a function of their ethical values and beliefs as it is of standards and compliance mechanisms' (Canadian Institute of Chartered Accountants 1997 page iv). The directors produce the culture of the organization, which in most businesses is the most powerful influence on the behaviour of the staff (Canadian Institute of Chartered Accountants 1997 para 40 Principle 4). ' "Control" comprises all the elements of an organisation (including its resources, systems, processes, culture, structure and tasks), which taken together, support people in the achievement of the organisation's objectives' (Canadian Institute of Chartered Accountants 1997 para 14). 'Control is as much a function of people's ethical values and beliefs as it is of standards and compliance mechanisms' (The Canadian Institute of Chartered Accountants 1999 Appendix A).

The control environment, therefore, provides the discipline and structure for the overall system of internal controls and generally includes such concerns as: integrity and ethical values of management; management's philosophy and operating style; organizational structure; assignment of authority and responsibility within the organization; human resources policies and practices; and competence of personnel hired within the organization. The board, therefore, has to set the culture of the organization to ensure that all employees understand the corporate purpose and are committed to delivering it (The Canadian Institute of Chartered Accountants 1999 page 2). The concern of the board must be to ensure that employees take risk knowingly, mitigate risk and strive to be prepared for the unknown. They must trust each other and communicate openly to get the job done, they must have the human, physical and financial resources required and they must monitor progress and adapt to new circumstances.

When all the components of culture, structure and processes are aligned and are as expected, this is the condition in which the organization is known to be 'in control'.

> The degree to which an organisation is in control is the result of all the interrelated elements that support its members in achieving corporate objectives. That is why conventional internal audit and risk management functions that address detailed procedures and individual risks are not sufficient to fulfil the directors' responsibilities in these areas. Whether an organisation is in control or not depends also on the elements as basic as the culture of the organisation, the adaptability and resourcefulness of its people and the calibre of its leadership.
> (The Canadian Institute of Chartered Accountants 1999 page 2)

Assurance and control

However, in the development of the concept of internal control as a tool of risk management (and as a result of auditors who could assess the internal control system but did not want to be held responsible for the outcome of the business), internal control became separated from the running of the business. Therefore, internal control was seen as a necessary support to but not a replacement for, good organizational management.

> Control does not constitute everything involved in managing an organisation. Control supports the achievement of reliable objectives: it does not tell people what objectives to set. Control can help ensure that the people responsible for monitoring and decision-making have appropriate, reliable information . . . Decisions about whether to act and what action to take are aspects of managing that are outside of control.
> (The Canadian Institute of Chartered Accountants 1995 Para 9 page 5)

As human behaviour can impact greatly on the success of an organisation, it is impossible for a board to guarantee that nothing will go wrong. There are inherent limitations in control. These include the possibilities of faulty judgement in decision making, breakdowns due to human error, control activities being circumvented by collusion of two or more people, and management overriding control (The Canadian Institute of Chartered Accountants 1995 page 3).

> Effective control is what makes an organisation reliable in achieving its objectives. Control is effective to the extent that it provides reasonable assurance that the organisation will achieve its objectives. Or, stated in another way, control is effective to the extent that the remaining risks of the organisation failing to meet its objectives are deemed acceptable.
>
> (Canadian Institute of Chartered Accountants 1997 para 14)

Therefore, boards are required to assure themselves that they have asked the right questions to reasonably assure themselves and their stakeholders that they have done the best they can, to achieve their organization's objectives by having effective internal controls. In turn, auditors are required to verify that boards have been effective in their assessment of internal control systems. Early control systems, based on concerns about financial impropriety, focused on detecting and preventing errors and irregularities from occurring (see table 3.2).

Additionally, cost benefit considerations can and should be taken into account when designing control in organizations. The costs of control must be balanced against the benefits, including the risks it is designed to manage. Design decisions involve the acceptance of some degree of risk: outcomes or actions cannot be predicted with absolute assurance (The Canadian Institute of Chartered Accountants 1995 page 3).

Table 3.2 Early definition of controls

Preventative controls are designed to discourage errors or irregularities from occurring. Example: Processing vouchers only after signatures have been obtained from appropriate personnel.

Detective controls uncover and correct undesirable events that have occurred. Detective controls should be designed to identify an error or irregularity after it has occurred. Reviewing long distance telephone charges for personal calls and preparing reconciliations are examples of detective controls.

Directive controls cause or encourage a desirable event to occur. Directive controls should be designed to assist in the accomplishment of goals and objectives. Training seminars and written job descriptions are examples of directive controls.

Human error and the concern about control resulted in a common theme emerging from these approaches to governance, which emphasized that the board and management of organizations can only be judged in terms of what is reasonable for a board to undertake in attempting to achieve its objectives – as opposed to guaranteeing success in achieving them. This is key to holding business organizations to account to their shareholders and stakeholders. It is not reasonable to expect boards to be able to predict all eventualities or changes in the external environment. But it is a function of their competence that they should be able to demonstrate that they were awake to possibilities of difficulties and future events and, where possible, had developed plans to mitigate risks or contingency plans to deal with likely futures. Furthermore, some organizations might exist to take risks and if so, stakeholders need to be confident that the organization understands risks and has made its stakeholders aware of the need to embrace risks.

The early approaches to the audit and, therefore, the production of assurance on internal control focused on those policies, procedures and management actions which ensured that the organization's assets were protected, records were accurate, operations were efficiently conducted and all policies, regulation and legislation were complied with. In order to provide assurance that management teams and organizations were achieving these aims, auditors developed a taxonomy of different types of controls which could be easily checked on. For example, they identified preventive, detective and directive controls (see table 3.2), which provided a framework for classifying controls and their associated risks for audit review. But this view presents control as a static set of structures within an organization and more recent thinking of control as a set of dynamic processes within an organisation could not accommodate this form of audit. Assurance demands that there are mechanisms for assessing control as a continuous process, rather than something that can be accounted for once a year. Although the Turnbull report called for boards to undertake a review of the effectiveness of their internal control system at least annually, the review of effectiveness was expected to be directed at demonstrating the existence of a robust and continuing process.

Auditors have, therefore, had to develop audit methodologies to help them identify internal control systems and the main models of internal control described above started their life as audit tools rather than management models. However, devising easy-to-use audit tools in this area is conceptually difficult. Audit checklists, which tried to assess the structural elements of internal control, have been tried in the USA and abandoned. After about six or seven years of struggling to use 'structure' when discussing internal control matters in audits of financial statements, the Auditing Standards Board decided to revert to the idea of internal control as a process rather than a structure and, therefore, to return to the model provided by COSO and the necessity to use a wide variety of tools to assess the effectiveness of internal control, while encompassing cultural issues. Checklists can be used to examine formal controls in organizations that use highly-structured processes but in cases where the organization depends more on individual or professional judgement, and softer informal controls are to be examined, auditors had to find other techniques that would address the culture of the organization.

Many consulting firms began to develop approaches to checking internal risk management as a method of providing assurance on internal control. This included the development of checklists for assessing the condition of organizations. This, it is argued, has given rise to a series of narrowing prescriptions put forward in models to be used by those who either do not fully understand all the implications, or who do not have the time to explore them (Mackay and Sweeting 2000). Care is needed in developing theoretical and rational approaches to organization-wide risk management, which are based around checklists, and far more understanding is required of the behavioural factors that managers bring with them in arriving at decisions and taking action (March 1987). External pressures on business organizations, such as the development of global competition, advances in information technology and what is referred to as 'the knowledge economy' have called for new approaches to management, which need to mobilize the creativity and discipline of all staff. This, in turn, has supported the requirement for a view of control based more on team working and culture than on prescribed processes (Canadian Institute of Chartered Accountants 1997 page iv).

One such technique, known as control self-assessment, is to encourage staff and managers to review the risks they face in their work and how these are managed. There are a number of ways this can be conducted, ranging from highly-interactive workshops based on behavioural models at one end of the spectrum to pre-packaged, self-audit, internal control questionnaires at the other end (McNamee 1996).

It has been suggested that there are six basic methods in use today, ranging from the most mechanical (least human contact), self-administered audit by Internal Control Questionnaire (ICQ) to the most behavioural (most human contact), such as group workshops (McNamee 1996). Internal Control Questionnaires are commonly used by external auditors to record their understanding of internal control. The ICQ is a series of questions used by the auditor as a checklist of expected controls. The questions are about various

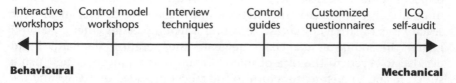

Figure 3.1   Control self-assessment continuum (from McNamee 1996).

control activities that may be or should be present in the operation. The ICQ is filled out by the auditor using observation and interviews during the preliminary assessment phase of the audit. The ICQ helps determine the level of control activity and, therefore, the level of testing and overall scope of the audit. This tool has been brought over and used successfully in traditional ('direct report') internal auditing as part of the preliminary survey phase of the internal audit. Some audit organizations take the ICQ and ask management to fill it out as a form of self-audit. Some auditors use this technique as a completed self-audit, while others use the results as a preliminary survey and risk assessment tool prior to an audit (McNamee 1996).

Auditors have, therefore, begun to recognize the importance of social or clan control in the delivery of good governance and organizational accountability. This required the development of auditing approaches and models for good governance that could embrace organizational culture, the developments in specialist working and concomitant teamworking while providing public accountability. It was becoming apparent to governments that regulation of corporate governance was neither manageable nor appropriate. Instead, encouraging disclosure of decision making and including open and transparent decision making as an integral part of the practice of corporate governance as opposed to merely listing good principles for good governance, was felt to be a better approach. 'Whilst there may be a place for regulating some aspects of corporate governance, our view is that disclosure is a much better approach than attempting to regulate behaviour if one is seeking to build a health governance culture' (Joint Committee on Corporate Governance 2001 page 10).

The government is responsible for the delivery of public services, which includes health care. Health care is dominated by professional groupings which, by definition, are social or clan groupings, who have evolved their own norms of behaviour which are not necessarily in tune with those of the wider public. The use of such behavioural tools is antithetical to most governmentally-determined views of health care, which currently are thought to demand less autonomy and more control from central government. However, governments have been accused of introducing too many controls into the management of public services including health care. Is it possible that these developments of thinking in the private business sector could have influenced public sector approaches to governance? And how could they contribute to improvements in the management and delivery of services such as health care? Is it possible that this could suggest how to achieve improvements of quality in health care and the assurance that individual patient care is held central to the governance of health services in the new structures of health care proposed under devolved management?

Chapter summary

This chapter has dealt with the following points:

* The balance between (de)regulation and accountability.
* The different approaches to corporate governance in various countries and how these approaches have been formalized.
* The implementation of internal controls through setting and achieving objectives, and assessing and dealing with risk, while providing methods of assurance.

4 The Modification of Internal Control: control in Government Departments

Governments are adept at developing social or societal control systems through the introduction of regulations. State regulation is defined as any government intervention or measure which controls, directs or restricts the behaviour of individuals (or organizations). The main purpose of regulation is to respond to and apply controls to minimize specific risks. 'Where individuals or businesses impose risks on others, government's role is mainly as regulator, setting the rules of the game' (Better regulation task force 2000a). This suggests that the rules of the game are the controls imposed on the behaviours of individuals or organizations, to reduce the risks that may be created for others. 'Where risks cannot be attributed to any specific individual or body, governments may take on a stewardship role to provide protection or mitigate the consequences' (Better regulation task force 2000a). Regulation, therefore, exists to protect individuals or society from risks which may harm the individual or the collective. With regard to the regulation of private sector activity, as shown in the previous chapter, it is generally claimed that businesses do not like regulation and prefer self-regulation because they fear external regulation will interfere with their activities. 'This, however, is the whole point of having external regulators. The idea is always to impose a certain shape on the market because, the assumption is, without regulation, the market will operate "unfairly" ' (Harrington 2002).

There has been acknowledgement of the need for a balance between controls and the resources they require and the desire to control risks (Department of Health 2001b; Interdepartmental Liaison Group on Risk Assessment 1998). However, although protection from risk is the main argument for regulation, there is little evidence of any correlation between levels of risk and the degree of state involvement in regulatory solutions. Rarely can it be shown that policy makers have used the degree of risk as a determining factor for deciding the level of state involvement in regulation (Better regulation task force 2000a page 8). In order to improve the process of creating regulations, the government established the Better regulation task force in September 1997, to advise the government on action that improves the effectiveness and credibility of government regulation by ensuring that it is necessary, fair, affordable and simple to understand and administer, taking particular account of the needs of small businesses and ordinary people.

The task force set out to test whether there was a correlation between state involvement and risk. They found that the schemes designed to regulate areas of greatest risk (accounting, medicine or legal services), rather than using direct state regulation in fact relied upon forms of self-regulation. The areas where official codes and state regulatory bodies (which they identified as the highest level of state involvement) proliferated were in areas that they felt were not particularly high risk, such as dispensing hearing aids and domestic telephone services (Better regulation task force 2000a para 3.3.3). They tried to rank different types of risk, albeit subjectively, and concluded that there was no logical explanation for the degree of regulation applied to different risks. They found that, for example, there was no reasonable explanation for why the regulations attached to employing a domestic builder, which would be relatively low risk, would be greater than those provided for the seeking of legal advice (Better regulation task force 2000a).

The government in the UK identified a set of general principles delimiting the areas where state regulation may be considered appropriate (see table 4.1). These focus on societal objectives, such as protecting the vulnerable; protecting and enhancing the rights and liberties of citizens; safeguarding health and safety; and promoting and protecting the environment. In addition, the Better regulation task force identified five principles for good regulation – transparency, proportionality, targeting, consistency and accountability (Better regulation task force 2000b).

Regulation and risk management

The 'big risks' to individual health and societal welfare were presenting increasingly difficult policy decisions for governments. The government was

Table 4.1 General principles for state regulation (Better regulation task force 2000b)

- Protect and enhance the rights and liberties of citizens.
- Promote a safe and peaceful society.
- Collect taxes and ensure that they are spent in accordance with policy objectives.
- Safeguard health and safety or protect citizens from 'harming' themselves.
- Protect consumers, employees and vulnerable groups from abuse.
- Promote the efficient working of markets.
- Protect the environment and promote sustainable development.

accused of lacking mechanisms for the anticipation of emerging risks to the public (Performance and Innovation Unit 2001b). These risks were recognized to require governmental control but, by their nature, presented considerable difficulties for governments in dealing with public expectations. As Powell and Leiss (1997) have shown in the case of mad cow disease, the failures of government to communicate with the public about high-profile risks have been seen to create considerable controversy and generate enormous and frequently unnecessary costs in regulation (Powell and Leiss 1997). Governments had also been accused of over-control with regard to issues affecting the public as much as they had for control of private businesses. The purpose of risk management and its consequent success for policy making was described as fewer surprises to the public and government, and better managed impact of unexpected events (less anxiety and panic, and lower costs); higher levels of safety and confidence (less loss of life and injury); and better understanding of risks and trade-offs between different options by public and government (for example, better decisions on pensions, smoking and diet) (Cabinet Office 2002).

The management of risks was key to successful government, heralding a new relationship between the government and the public. The Modernisation Action Plan produced in 1999, as a main plank of the then Labour government's policy agenda, required all departments to make public the framework and procedures they use for reaching decisions on the risks for which they are responsible. The desire for increased accountability was addressed in the field of regulation by increasing the extent of ministerial and parliamentary scrutiny of regulation, and subsequent evaluation of whether regulation achieved its intended objectives (National Audit Office 2001b). Each proposed regulation would be assessed using a technique known as Regulatory Impact Assessment, intended to enable the public to understand what a proposed regulation was trying to achieve and to challenge the assumptions upon which it was based. The accountability argument upon which this development was based was that, in making regulatory frameworks publicly available, the public should have better knowledge and a greater ability to question rules being created on their behalf (National Audit Office 2001c).

In addition, the government had undertaken to produce a public declaration on the management of risk, which eventually appeared in late 2002. This was all part of a European move to harmonize risk assessment and a recognition that the government needed to look to other countries to learn lessons on risk management and to integrate with European and international dimensions in public policy. In 2000, the first report on the harmonization of risk assessment procedures (Working group on harmonization of risk assessment procedures in the scientific committees advising the European Commission in the area of human and environmental health 2000) called for active debate on current practices for risk assessment used by the commission's scientific committees and to make proposals for developing convergent approaches that will aid harmonization across the EC. The breadth of risk was recognized. 'A risk assessment is required for increasing numbers of human activities, ranging from the prognoses for mental health patients, through industrial plant safety to sensitive ecological sites and consumer protection' (Working group on harmonization of risk assessment procedures in the scientific committees advising the European Commission in the area of human and environmental health 2000 para 2.1). This is risk as defined in terms of hazard, which can cause harm to individuals or populations. Hazards tend to be described using scientific evidence to denote the uncertainties attached to doing harm which, in turn, tend to persuade the general public of their validity. This has led governments to develop increasingly scientific approaches to the assessment of risk and the specification of associated standards (HM Treasury 1997). Activities for which new proposals need to be appraised include specification of standards such as the choice of standards for health and safety, or for environmental quality or sustainability; or for the insulation, fire protection, lighting or design of buildings; or to balance compliance costs with the benefits of regulation.

Most of the thinking about risk had evolved in dealing with hazards in businesses and this did not translate adequately into thinking about policy making or service delivery. To accommodate the wide variety of risks faced by government departments, an attempt was made to identify two different styles of risk management to be used in government. One was called 'anticipation' – identifying risks in advance and putting in place measures to prevent those risks, or at least reduce their probability or severity; and 'resilience' – creating generic organizational capability for flexible response when harms, costs and obstacles do fall (Performance and Innovation Unit 2001b Para 13). It is the development of the anticipation risk approach that has caused the most difficulty in policy making and management.

Where there are statistical data, it is possible to produce information on the probabilities of events occurring and risks can be quantified. But in public policy there is considerable uncertainty about what action to take and how to measure outcome, often deriving from lack of information. As noted earlier, two types of uncertainty were identified as of concern for government. Uncertainty that comes from lack of information needs to be handled differently from uncertainty that derives from the unpredictability of events. Lack of information in risk management is not ignorance, which occurs when hazards have not been fully identified and there is a lack of data. Uncertainty in policy terms is a concern when scientific and statistical robustness cannot be tested. There is, for example, an international agreement to apply what is known as the Precautionary Principle, which exists to rule out the lack of certain scientific evidence as a reason for not taking preventive action (Le Guen 1999 page 31). The Precautionary Principle describes the philosophy that should be adopted for addressing risks subject to high uncertainty, particularly in the environmental field. It is incorporated in the EEC Treaty under article 120r and other international treaties and conventions concerned with global environmental issues, e.g. climate change (Interdepartmental group on risk assessment 2002). Though not defined in the EEC treaty, the Precautionary Principle has been defined by the United Nations Conference on the Environment and Development (UNCED) in 1992 as: 'Where there are threats of serious or irreversible environmental damage lack of full scientific certainty shall not be used as a reason for postponing cost effective measure to prevent degradation' (Cabinet Office 2001). Therefore, where there is enough evidence for believing a hazard to exist, action should be taken to prevent its harmful effects. It has not been easy to implement this approach as there has been considerable confusion in government departments as to how to interpret it. (Interdepartmental Liaison Group on Risk Assessment 1998 chapter 3 page 5). In many areas of public policy, even that which might at first appear to be certain is not always as well grounded in scientific certainty and objectivity as the general public would wish to believe.

> Regulators have traditionally sought legitimacy for their decisions by wrapping them in a cloak of scientific respectability. Their determinations (they claim) are firmly based on scientific analyses made by qualified experts. But the cognitive and institutional complexity of pollution control and risk evaluation has dispelled the initial faith in the power of such experts. The scientific and conceptual basis of environmental regulation is so precarious, the empirical evidence so ambiguous, that most regulatory decisions can only be evaluated and legitimated in terms of procedural, rather than substantive, rationality – by process not by outcome.
>
> (Majone 1983 page 307)

In the absence of full evidence, it was decided to base decisions on risk assessment using a precautionary approach and to build the anticipation of risks into the strategic management of government departments. 'Strategic decision making where uncertainty is high, the approach to risk management will tend to rely on exploring scenarios, past experience of generic hazards and analysis of whether action needs to be taken to avoid serious consequences of very uncertain events' (Cabinet Office 2002; Performance and Innovation Unit 2001b para 19). However, high levels of uncertainty and lack of precision in the definition and measurement of risk mean that any perceived risk is highly subjective and it is not possible to supply adequate evidence to the public on the impact or likelihood of risks. Therefore, given that the role of government is to protect the public, the government must respond to public perceptions of risk if is it is to be accountable for its actions with regard to regulation.

> It is now widely accepted that managing risks solely on the basis of probabilistic estimate of physical harm is unlikely to succeed. Public values and perceptions of risk must also be integrated in the decision making process, though how these can be taken into account in any particular case will depend on constraints (such as the EC or international obligations) . . .
> (Interdepartmental Liaison Group on Risk Assessment 1998 chapter 3 para 3)

Internationally, government policy was acknowledging that ideas about risk are shaped by social experience as much as they are by scientific inquiry (Government of Victoria 2000). As a consequence, it was felt to be necessary to involve as many groups and views as possible in the assessments of risk and the solutions considered and decided upon, to ensure that these solutions are acceptable to as many stakeholders as possible. Slovik (2002) has pointed out that while recognizing interested citizens as legitimate partners in the exercise of risk assessment is no short-term panacea for the problem of risk management, it is possible that paying serious attention to participation in the process may, in the longer term, lead to more successful ways to manage risks.

The government also had to ensure that, with the new emphasis on accountability, the public understood that risk management is not a precise science, particularly if the public were involved in the assessment of risks. Decision making can go wrong and not all risks can be eradicated: 'with perseverance, it should be possible to persuade the media and the public that an essential aspect of good government is to take risks on our behalf recognising that, with the best will in the world, some will fail' (Better regulation task force 2000b page 6). In the UK this resulted in government recognition of the need to improve decision making, making sure evidence is well grounded and where it is not, there is clear consultation on risks, which responds to and recognizes public concerns. This was essential to building the much needed trust and to do this, decisions had to reflect public attitudes and values, which required a more proactive and two-way communication process. 'In a free and democratic society, where Ministers are accountable to Parliament, and thereby, to the public, societal values and the public's willingness to accept or tolerate risk are relevant and legitimate considerations for public decision-making, whether or not they are consistent with a scientific assessment of the risk' (Report of the ADM working group on risk management 2000 page 4). Trust was also felt to be crucial in obtaining acceptance of risk management decisions and mistrust laid at the root of conflicts about the validity of risk assessments and decisions made on them.

> We know that trust is not automatically bestowed, we also know that the Government can earn that trust by ensuring, amongst other

things, that Departments and their Agencies have consistent, fair and transparent approaches that reflect the values of society.

(Interdepartmental Liaison Group on Risk Assessment 1998 chapter 3 para 4)

It was rapidly recognized that the subjective nature of risk would mean that resulting policy solutions would vary according to the perspective applied. All risk assessment is laden with subjective judgements and different groups of people perceive risk differerntly (Slovic 2002). Studies in the 1970s had shown that hazards about which people have little knowledge were feared as being the most risky. The public was also found to have very different views about risk from the experts. There was a recognition by governments that the nature of the risk assessment had to broaden but, in turn, it was felt that the public should have: more realistic expectations of the government's ability to protect them from risk; greater recognition of the expectations and responsibilities of individuals to manage the risks that affect them directly; and better information that enables individuals to form balanced judgements about the scale and the likelihood of risks and the choice of response. The Cabinet Office, therefore, promoted greater stakeholder engagement in policy development to improve the perception of risk to all those involved in a policy (Public Accounts Committee 2001 para 14), in order to advance the modernization agenda (Cabinet Office 1999 page 16).

Public involvement

Particularly in areas that affected public safety, there was a need for the information made available to the public to be more relevant and up-to-date, plus greater clarity about the assumptions underpinning any decisions, particularly where there was uncertainty, a lack of information or conflicting views (Public Accounts Committee 2002). This was considered necessary to improve public trust in central government decision making. The Better regulation task force's fourth annual report suggested that trust is more likely to be strong where:

Institutions are clear about their objectives and values; there is openness and transparency around decisions; decisions are clearly grounded in evidence; public values and concerns are taken into account in making decisions; sufficient information is provided to allow individuals to make balanced judgements; and mistakes are quickly acknowledged and acted on.

(Cabinet Office 2002 page 76)

These principles call for more systematic involvement of the public in the decisions that affect them, requiring communication to start early in the policy development and decision process. A major concern was to prevent the unintended consequences of new regulations. It was suggested that there should be more creativity in the selection of people who are to be consulted and finding better ways of involving them in consultation exercises. It was also suggested that there should be specific questions on whether consultees could see any unintended adverse effects on specific groups. The UK government had suffered particularly from the introduction of minimum standards for care homes for the elderly, which although intended to improve quality had been found to be too expensive to implement, resulting in the unintended consequence of the closure of a number of homes (Better regulation task force 2000b). Departments were criticized for tending to consult a usual list of contacts, who were vulnerable to what was described as 'group think'. To prevent key risks from being missed, it was proposed that the list of contacts to be consulted should be widened.

Government departments were not enthusiastic about the demands for increased consultation and expressed concern about what they called 'consultation fatigue' if they were required to go repeatedly to too many members of the public and stakeholders. In particular, they were concerned about the need to consult on risks relating to internal management of their business. The response was an attempt to focus risk assessment on the handling of risks that affect the public directly, such as health, property, investments or the environment. These public issues required the creation of policy, and risk in this activity was, therefore, categorized under four main headings: actual risk; communication risk; policy process risk; and loss of capacity to make policy.

There were also concerns about risks that were shared between government departments and how these should be handled. There was an emerging view in Canada that horizontal risk management, that is, elements of risk and procedures for dealing with risk which are common to various government policy responsibilities should be identified across government departments to develop a coherent process of dealing with uncertainty within a public policy environment (Report of the ADM working group on risk management 2000 page 2).

For the management of the internal business of running departments, government departments preferred to look for a method that would enable them to handle risks in a less public way. The preference was to adopt the view of risk management associated with internal control as portrayed in the Turnbull report, which was adopted in full by government departments. The strategy unit of the Cabinet Office, therefore, recommended that systematic approaches to strategic policy making should be introduced, which should be adapted to recognize the less quantifiable nature of the data involved (Cabinet Office 2002 para 4.2.40). This required a subjective assessment of risk derived from a subjective assessment of the likelihood of an event or hazard occurring and combining this with a subjective assessment of the severity or the importance of the risk. In some areas such as health and safety, there is a need to reduce the risk to levels that are as low as reasonably practical. In other areas, the risks can be assessed to identify their relative priority, and the urgency with which they should be acted upon.

Government management of projects

The Cabinet Office was made responsible for encouraging departments to adopt well-managed risk taking where it was likely to lead to sustainable improvements in service delivery. But the civil service was felt to believe that risk taking was associated with increasing the possibility of things going wrong, which would lead to parliamentary censure and damage to personal careers (Strategic policy making team, Cabinet Office 1999 para 5.35). The experience of government in handling risks had demonstrated significant gaps in the ability of government departments to understand risk and to manage it (Cabinet Office 2002 page 9). The National Audit Office report had noted that the absence of early warning indicators led to key risks to service delivery not being identified, or being identified too late, for effective action to be taken to remedy the situation (Performance and Innovation Unit 2001b para 16). The Modernising Government programme, which focuses on sustainable improvements in service delivery, actively encouraged the public sector to adopt risk taking in order to innovate in service design and delivery – and so in taking risks, the public sector needs to undertake risk management.

> The cultures of Parliament, Ministers and the civil service create a situation in which the rewards for success are limited and penalties for failure can be severe. The system is too often risk averse. As a result, Ministers and public servants can be slow to take advantage of new opportunities.
>
> (Cabinet Office 1999 page 11)

For project management conducted by government departments, the cabinet office suggested successful outcomes should be judged in terms of such things as fewer direct costs resulting from failure to anticipate risks – for example, from failed projects such as the Passport Office processing system (£12.6 million) or Benefits Payment Card (£127 million) – and a better balance of risk and opportunity. Good risk management can provide the confidence necessary for taking innovative decisions (limiting risk through pilots or careful management of project risks) (Cabinet Office 2002). The Cabinet Office had accepted the dominant corporate governance view that improvements in risk management would lead to higher levels of performance by departments and would reduce the likelihood of major failures in service delivery (Public Accounts Committee 2001).

> All activity by government departments involves the risk that projects or programmes may fail, that services may not be delivered on time or to a satisfactory standard, or that opportunities may be missed. Assessment of the likelihood of such contingencies arising is essential if departments are to take decisions on the basis of best information and thus maximize the likelihood of being able to meet their objectives . . . Numerous reports by this Committee have emphasized the need for departments to improve their risk management. In particular we have drawn attention to the importance of departments undertaking careful risk assessments before embarking on major new projects and programmes of having strategies for managing risks, and of having reliable contingency arrangements in place for responding to the unexpected, so that service delivery for citizens can be maintained.
>
> (Public Accounts Committee 2001 paras 1 and 2)

Part of the argument behind better risk management is to increase or enhance what is referred to as the 'risk appetite' of organizations, particularly boards. Organizations need to innovate, and to innovate they must be prepared to take risks. There was, therefore, a move to advance the definition of risk to include opportunity, a move similar to that which had taken place in the private sector. 'There is considerable debate and discussion on what would be an acceptable generic definition of risk that would recognize the fact that, when assessed and managed properly, risk can lead to innovation and opportunity. This situation appears to be more prevalent when dealing with operational risks and in the context of technological risks' (Treasury Board of Canada 2000 page 4). Therefore, the public sector organization must be encouraged to become less fearful of getting things wrong. Fear of failing to deliver and fear of auditors who criticized risk taking was felt to have instilled a culture of risk aversion into the public services (Lord Sharman 2002).

Government departments were also considered to be incapable of making investment and programme management decisions appropriately because of their inability to handle risk properly. On the one hand, they were considered to be too risk averse, failing to take new opportunities for improvement. On the other hand, where government departments did make changes, they were criticized for poor risk management. 'Too often central government does not assess the risk and walks off the end of a cliff. It does not consider where it is going and when it marches forward it does not manage the risk. Too often, there are no pilot projects, no training and no contingency plans' (Sir John

Bourn 2002 para 5.33). Government bodies are responsible for a broad range of activities, many of which involve a degree of risk (Lord Sharman 2002 para 5.33). More recently, however, the growth of new forms of service delivery, such as under the Private Finance Initiative, has highlighted the importance of identifying key risks and allocating responsibility for managing them to the most appropriate party. The Modernizing Government programme took as its central platform the need to encourage departments to adopt well-managed risk taking where it can lead to sustainable improvements in service (Lord Sharman 2002 Para 5.34).

The Cabinet Office were given responsibility for encouraging departments to adopt well-managed risk taking where it was likely to lead to sustainable improvements in service delivery. To this end, government departments were asked to produce and publish on their websites plans for handling those risks for which they are responsible that could directly affect the public, in particular health, safety and environmental risks (Public Accounts Committee 2001 para 5). 'Risk management has been defined as a corporate and systematic process for evaluating and addressing the impact of risks in a cost effective way and having staff with the appropriate skills to identify and assess the potential for risks to arise' (National Audit Office 2000 Para 5.37).

However, there was growing concern that departments were focusing only on the better known risks, such as safety hazards and risks associated with scientific uncertainty. The survey of departments by the National Audit Office found that their approach to risk management was focused on minimizing financial loss or preventing impropriety (National Audit Office 2000). There was, however, less recognition by departments that risk management is also about ensuring the achievement of outputs and outcomes and having reliable contingency arrangements to deal with the unexpected, which might put service delivery at risk. The Public Accounts Committee's report on the passport delays of the summer of 1999 highlighted a clear example of where service delivery was significantly at risk and where contingency arrangements had not been established to minimize the adverse impact on service delivery for the public (Public Accounts Committee 1999). The Cabinet Office had a number of initiatives underway to ensure that risk management covered all aspects of departments' business from policy development to managing projects and service delivery on the ground. These initiatives included reviewing departments' risk frameworks with the assistance of independent consultants to identify good practice and areas requiring improvement; working with the Treasury to improve the quarterly monitoring of how well departments are meeting their public service agreements; and service delivery agreement targets and seminars on risk management between ministers and officials.

Internal control methods

The response to the identified need for improved risk management was the seeking of improved control systems. Control was interpreted as the need to contain the uncertainty of outcome that has been identified in relation to any action, procedure or operation undertaken by management, thereby increasing the likelihood that activities and procedures achieve their objectives (HM Treasury 2001 para 4.2.42). The ideas from the audit literature were re-interpreted for government departments. Detective controls, such as after-the-event assessments including evaluations and post implementation reviews, were felt to be increasingly routinely applied. Directive and preventive controls, which covered specific risk mitigation measures, were aimed at ensuring that particular outcomes were achieved or preventing the possibility of an undesirable outcome being realized. It was claimed that use and monitoring of such measures was becoming more widespread. Corrective controls, which were identified as correcting already experienced undesirable outcomes, included crisis management arrangements and the contingency planning that underpins them. These were identified as areas where recent events had highlighted a need for attention and better approaches at the highest levels of government.

The Treasury suggested two main approaches that could be adopted for the identification of operational risk (HM Treasury 2001). The first was commissioning a risk review in which a designated team is established (either in-house or contracted in) to consider all the operations and activities of the organization in relation to its objectives and to identify the associated risks. It was suggested that the team should work by conducting a series of interviews with key staff at all level of the organization, to build a risk profile for the whole range of activities. The second approach was entitled 'risk self-assessment', which aimed to be a bottom up approach by which each level and part of the organization is invited to review its activities and to feed upwards its diagnosis of the risks faced. This may be done through a documentation approach (with a framework for diagnosis set out through questionnaires) or through a facilitated workshop approach (using facilitators with appropriate skills to help groups of staff to work out the risks affecting their areas of responsibility).

The identification of risks generated from operational activities, a bottom-up approach to risk identification, led to concerns about the need to record risks for accountability purposes (see Table 4.2). This was part of the acceptance of central government that there was a need to make all risks explicit. However this need, combined with concerns that there were no systematic and structured ways of dealing with risks employed in government departments, was felt to undermine accountability. There was no auditable trail of judgements about risks which made it impossible to review risk judgements.

Table 4.2 Steps in the risk management process (Cabinet Office 2002)

- Risks have to be identified and assessed, with responsibility and accountability allocated and clear.
- Judgement is needed about their importance.
- Mitigation and contingency plans may need to be considered.
- The impact of actions on risks needs to be reviewed and reported.
- Information and decisions need to be effectively communicated.

And this created difficulties for departments when held to account by the Public Accounts Committee. It was clear that operational risks did not demonstrate improved handling of government objectives. It was decided that a systematic approach was required at every level of decision making, that is: strategic, programme and operational. Although these levels have distinct characteristics, a common model to approach risk assessment was felt to be possible for use across central government, thereby providing the necessary move towards the standardization of risk assessment desired by the proponents of integrated risk management. The ensuing guidance contained clear directions about the significant elements of risk handling by government departments in which a primary concern was the demonstration of accountability. Key features were the allocation of responsibility and accountability for risk identification and assessment, with the ability to make judgements about their importance (Cabinet Office 2002).

The need to record risks generated interest in the creation of a register of risks to record and compare risks within and across government departments. However, no clear advice or single model has been produced on the construction of a risk register. In some models, the risk register collects all risks and synthesizes them to identify significant risks that need to be passed to the board. In other models, the content of the risk register is restricted to only those items that relate to the significant strategic risks identified by the board as fundamental to its objectives. 'There must be sufficient information to make it worthwhile collating the information but each organisation will need to decide its own content requirements for each entry' (Office of Government Commerce 2002 chapter 8 page 54).

Integrated or organization-wide risk management requires that risks of very different types are compared and prioritized, so that the board can be alerted to the most significant risks that should warrant their attention. The most commonly used methodology for comparing risks of a very different nature is a risk matrix, which plots a single, ascribed value of probability against a single, ascribed value of consequence and, therefore, reduces risk to a single, easily comparable value (albeit based on a purely subjective judgement). The matrix is a form of presentation (a single table); which enables easy comparison of the values placed on different risks (Garvey and Landowne 2004). The purpose of systematically assigning values to risks is to create a standardized approach to the assignment of probability and consequence, applied to all risks across the organization which, in theory, should minimize the variation in the judgements applied to risks across the organization (Health care standards unit and the risk management working group 2004). Once the risks are reduced to the same value on this scale, it is possible to consider the issues involved in managing the risks and to prioritize them in order of need for action (see Table 4.3).

However, there are well recognized difficulties with this approach. 'We are taught we should not compare apples with pears. Yet in ranking risks we may be faced with comparing peas with planets. Society is not yet evolved to the point where it is able to deal with the ethical issues that arise when comparisons are made between different kinds of risks' (Interdepartmental Liaison Group on Risk Assessment 1998 chapter 3 page 6). A survey of government departments found that many were attempting to develop taxonomies which would enable them to populate a risk register and thereby manage the variety and complexity of risks by developing short, grouped lists of risks but that there was no single coherent approach to classifying risks. As there was no single standardized approach to classifying and assessing risks, this meant they could not be compared and prioritized across government departments. In addition, the lack of a common categorization of risks hindered communication about risks across government. As a consequence, it was recommended that risks within central government should be categorized as strategic (including major external threats, significant cross-cutting risks, and longer-term

Table 4.3 Risk profile matrix
Qualitative risk analysis matrix – level of risk

Likelihood	Consequences Insignificant 1	Minor 2	Moderate 3	Major 4	Catastrophic 5
A (almost certain)	H	H	E	E	E
B (likely)	M	H	H	E	E
C (moderate)	L	M	H	E	E
D (unlikely)	L	L	M	H	E
E (rare)	L	L	M	H	H

Legend: E: extreme risk; immediate action required.
     H: high risk; senior management attention needed.
     M: moderate risk; management responsibility must be specified.
     L: low risk; manage by routine procedures.
(from Health care standards unit and the risk management working group 2004).

threats and opportunities); and delivery (including both operational and project/programme risks) (Office of Government Commerce 2002). This simple and broad approach reflected the growing view that although some risks may be more difficult to assess than others (such as the macro economic changes or the delivery of objectives by second-tier or partner organizations), the assessment and prioritization process in these highly subjective areas of risk assessment should not be a complex exercise. 'Risk management is not rocket science – key risks are being managed albeit informally all the time by all organisations' (QUEST 2000 para 7 page 24).

The Office of Government Commerce attempted to unravel this complexity by identifying different types of management which require different approaches to risk. They recognized the need for clearly stated strategic objectives – 'without a clear view of the strategic objectives and goals, risk analysis and management may be inappropriately applied at all levels of the organisation. Commitments to corporate governance are made at this level' (Office of Government Commerce 2002 page 33). Middle-level managers, which the Office of Government Commerce recognized have the most difficult task, are responsible for transforming high-level strategy into politically acceptable solutions. These managers are typically responsible for a number of projects. The risk and opportunity trade-offs involved become even more complex as projects compete with one another for resources. The middle- or programme-level managers are primarily responsible for identifying and detailing solutions to conflicts associated with the implementation of strategic plans over which they have little influence. In addition, programme-level managers have to act as 'fire fighters' – responsible for keeping specific project crises from getting out of control and affecting the strategic objectives of the organization. To help deal with concerns at this level, programme-level managers will have the strategic-level risk policy that sets down processes, procedures and roles and responsibilities for use across the organization. At the project level, risk management focuses on keeping unwanted outcomes to the minimum. Finally, risk management at the operational level is primarily concerned with continuity of business services (Office of Government Commerce 2002 page 43). Operational managers are 'aiming to deliver a product or service, day after day, week after week after week. The manager must focus on the risk of not being able to provide the product or service to an adequate level of quality' (Office of Government Commerce 2002 page 47).

Using objectives in strategic risk management

The Office of Government Commerce suggested that the management of risk at the strategic or corporate level was concerned with setting strategic direction and balancing potential opportunity against the costs and risks.

Good appraisal entails being clear about objectives, thinking about alternative ways of meeting them, estimating and presenting the costs and benefits of each potentially worthwhile option and taking full account of associated risks and uncertainties. Good evaluation, after the event, entails many of the same demands together with a desire and willingness to look for better decisions by policy makers and managers.

(HM Treasury 1997 para 1.1)

Strategic risk meant examining the widest context of the business: 'its financial, legislative, political, social, competitive and cultural environments' (Office of Government Commerce 2002 page 33). The report suggested that this sort of analysis is intuitive in nature and, therefore, a formal approach to the identification of risk is required. Formality, it was held, would lead to high quality decision making. 'In addition, if a formal analysis approach is adopted, the information on risks identified at this level can be passed down the organisation for further analysis and resolution' (Office of Government Commerce 2002 page 34). The assumption being that formal analysis of the setting of objectives was accepted by the HM Treasury and other departments.

The focus on strategic risks in meeting governmental and departmental objectives brought with it the idea of limiting risk identification and assessment to those areas which impact on strategic risk, just as the idea had developed for private businesses. It was agreed that the objectives should be kept to a manageable number – the Orange Book recommended no more than ten (HM Treasury 2000b). The focus of risk identification should be restricted to those risks that might impact on, either positively or negatively, the achievement of strategic objectives (QUEST 2000). This would restrict the number of key risks to be identified as relevant to these objectives to a manageable number. Indeed, the advice suggested that the risk identification process could also serve to validate the setting of strategic objectives – 'if risks are identified that have no relation to the strategic objective a review of objectives should be triggered' (QUEST 2000 para 7 page 23).

The strategy unit report also recommended that there should be a combination of top-down and bottom-up approaches, 'for example combining a risk review (external assessment by senior management or a designated team) with risk self-assessment (by those directly involved), feeding up diagnosis of risk through the levels of the organisation' (Cabinet Office 2002 4.2.23). The Treasury guidance recommended that 'appropriate awareness of, and responsibility for risk issues lies in parallel with the structure of objectives. At every level of objectives there should be a parallel delegation of responsibility for the associated risk issues' (H.M. Treasury 2000b para 9.1). The assigning of ownership to identified risk was critical to the success of the risk management process. Some departments are organized with management boards, emulating the private sector structures, and in these boards members were felt to be learning how to take ownership of strategic risks, and so identifying individual members to act as risk owners on behalf of the board promoted personal responsibility. The Cabinet Office cited one department as having succeeded in producing a list of 12 top threats, which were selected using agreed criteria for senior action, and this department had assigned the management of these threats to individuals. Another department was reported to have created a strong dialogue between its board and Ministers on the handling of key risks. But in spite of good practice starting to emerge, it was still the case that risk management systems lagged behind those of financial management in terms of accountability and responsibility (Cabinet Office 2002).

The identification of objectives and strategic risk pointed the way to moving from the view of risk management as concerned with liabilities to something which would speak to vision and opportunities. It was recognized in some departments that companies had been successful in integrating environmental and safety risk and control with other business areas, such as fraud and information technology. This, it was argued, enabled management systems to be dealt with in a strategic way, which could emphasize employee involvement; but concerns still existed that formalized risk management could still reduce innovation and the willingness to take risks. There were, therefore, attempts to devise approaches to risk management which would fit into business planning processes rather than following the parallel approach recommended by the Treasury (Wheeler & Silanpaa 1997).

It was anticipated that the focus on strategic risk would evolve as organizations mature in their understanding of the requirements for establishing internal control (Cabinet Office 2002). The preoccupation of audit with protection from hazards would be replaced by line managers evaluating and managing risks to operating performance. As the organization matures, the focus of risk assessment and management should move to the strategic issues facing the organization, this move would be led by the board and senior management (see Figure 4.1)

The recognition of the need for better risk management, combined with the influence of the Turnbull report, led to requirements for government departments to produce assurances on their internal controls. 'Reliable controls can minimize the likelihood of risks maturing, for example by preventing unauthorized use of expenditure or by highlighting deficiencies in the quality of a service and can mininize the adverse consequences if a risk does mature' (Public Accounts Committee 2001 para 6). Guidance for departments on internal controls is the responsibility of the Treasury, which is seeking to apply to central government departments the principles of the Turnbull report (Public Accounts Committee 2001 para 6). In 1997, UK government departments were required by the Treasury to produce a statement on Internal Financial Control (HM Treasury 2000a), which, in effect, introduced the

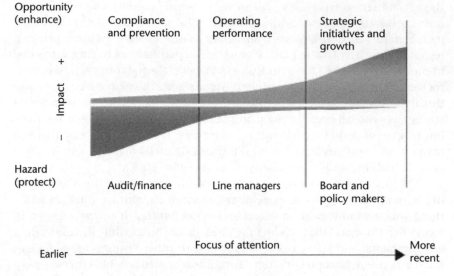

Figure 4.1 Typical development of risk management within an organisation (from Cabinet Office 2003).

concepts of financial governance into the reporting of public sector accounts. Following the Turnbull report, the Treasury determined to introduce the same wider provisions on internal control into the public sector which were contained in a Treasury letter of 22nd December 2000 (HM Treasury 2000a). This required each department to produce a Statement on Internal Control to be presented alongside the accounts of the department. Based on the words of Turnbull, the letter requires that the Statement on Internal Control should be 'the end result of a process of management that is embedded in the planning, operational, monitoring and review activities of the body'. The insistence that the production of the Statement of Internal Control should not be seen as an add-on, end-of-year activity confirmed the view that this was to be a part of a whole management process incorporated into every government department.

The Treasury is required under the Government Resources and Accounts Act 2000 and the Government Trading Funds Act 1973 to appoint an accounting officer in each government department and trading fund. Additional accounting officers may also be appointed in departments and accounting officers are designated in the vast majority of executive agencies and non departmental public bodies. By convention, the head of the organization, in the case of a government department the Permanent Secretary, is appointed as its accounting officer to report to parliament on the conduct of the business of the department and to sign off the accounts of the organization (HM Treasury 2002a para 2.2).

The purpose of the Statement of Internal Control (SIC) was, therefore, to encourage an emphasis on strategic risk management rather than operational risk management. 'These will be premised on strategic risk management processes embedded in the operation of the organisation' (Office of Government Commerce 2002 para 1.3). The National Audit Office's review of departmental SICs is an assessment of whether the audited body's description of the processes adopted in reviewing the effectiveness of the system of internal control appropriately reflects those processes. Work for this includes: attendance at audit committee meetings at which corporate governance, internal control and risk management matters are considered; consideration of whether disclosures to parliament and the public made by the department are consistent with knowledge obtained by the National Audit Office during its audit work; and consideration of how well accounting officers have conducted their effectiveness reviews (National Audit Office 2002 para 3.46).

> All central government bodies should follow the private sector in applying the principles of the Turnbull report as a basis for ensuring strong internal controls and management within the process of government. The discipline of having a formal internal control statement, signed by the accounting officer, is helping departments to systematize and, where necessary, overhaul their internal controls systems. To be able to sign the statement, the Accounting Officer will need to take assurance from other senior staff that proper systems and controls are in place. Given this, the Accounting Officer's statement should make clear he has placed reliance on these assurances. This will ensure that the overall accountability of the Accounting Officer is maintained, whilst making clear the responsibilities of other senior officials.
>
> (Lord Sharman 2002 Recommendation 1)

Following this, the Treasury announced its intention to clarify the accounting officer's responsibilities for risk management, control and governance through the restatement of the anouncement on internal control. It also announced the intention to further clarify the methods by which risks would be managed by central government (HM Treasury 2002a Para 3.45).

The government and its departments had, therefore, accepted the significance of risk management and, by association, the importance of controls within the organization and the management of government departments. This demonstrated a commitment to follow the Turnbull requirements to implement organisation-wide risk management and control systems and by so doing would make departments more accountable for the policy-making process. However, it was not clear that this would lead to direct improvements in the delivery of the outcomes of public services. This required an additional dimension to be added to the delivery of public services, namely the introduction of precisely articulated desired outcomes, while at the same time reducing the extent of the direct management of services.

The senior levels of government departments are, therefore, required to behave in a manner similar to the boards of companies. Where they deal with issues concerning the protection of the public they face great uncertainties in scientific knowledge and in outcomes. Therefore, they are required to consult with the public to ensure the public understands the approaches to the management of risk adopted by government. But government departments are also involved in their own day-to-day management. The logic of implementing Turnbull requires that they understand the controls that exist in their own departments. But more importantly, they also run projects and provide services. And where innovation is required in the provision of service, they are required to understand the risks inherent in often large-scale project management. This requires processes to ensure that government departments are able to deliver the promised outcomes of new services, new schemes and new buildings. They, therefore, need to have operational risk management built into their processes. But where they deal with organizations over which they do not have direct control, there is a need to implement a more devolved method of promoting assurance based on risk management.

Chapter Summary

This chapter has dealt with the following points:

- What are appropriate levels of state regulation in the management of risks.
- The involvement of the public and government in risk management.
- Using different methods of internal control to assess risk.
- Using objectives in strategic risk management.

5 Standardizing internal control: controls in the National Health Service

The desire to devolve power to organizations has meant that there is a need for the government to reduce direct control over organizations but an increased, counter-balancing need to ensure that independent organizations conform to the vision and values set by government. As direct management control reduces, so the desire to regulate increases.

> Governments have been keen to divorce themselves from the direct provision of services. In so doing they have created the need to check that organisations operating in the name of government, whether publicly or privately owned are acting in the best interests of individuals and society at large. The growth of new Public Management (that is decentralisation of decision makers to public service managers) is based upon the assumption that governments should regulate and not manage services. However, responsibility for management without direct control generates greater concerns for regulation. It tends to be the case that core government departments are not subjected to as much regulation as outer departments. The further the service is from direct control the greater the degree of regulation the civil service tends to impose upon it.
>
> (Vass and Simmonds 2001a p11)

The proliferation of review bodies is the product of what has been termed 'mirror-imaging' – the tendency to create control bodies whenever authority is devolved (Hood *et al*. 1999; Vass and Simmonds 2001b).

Regulation includes the 'authorization' or 'registration' of bodies to undertake regulated activities and the monitoring of their compliance with statutory requirements and professional standards. It may also include prescription of compulsory activities and price controls (Public Audit Forum 2001). The main reason for regulation in the public sector is to ensure that the activities of organizations are controlled, because although governments are not directly managing organizations, the fact that they are still in government ownership means that any damage caused by these organizations to either individual members of the public, communities or, possibly, the financial stability of the government would still be laid at the government's door. The focus of accountability, therefore, is located where the public perceives the responsibility for the control of services to lie. For devolution to work, there has to be a transfer of ownership from central government to the management of services, but equally there has to be public recognition that the relocation of ownership also creates a relocation of accountability.

An argument in favour of reducing central regulation is that, although the role of central government may be to structure a regulatory environment to protect society from broad risks, it tends not to have the expertise to devise formal control systems for the direct management of services. In fact, it would be surprising if this were the case, for central government departments are effective machinery for the production and implementation of ministerial policies. But as earlier chapters have demonstrated, quality of health care is a complex phenomenon, and cannot be driven solely through political aspirations for parts of the system. It would indeed be surprising if civil servants were trained and knowledgeable about the systems required to run individual health care organizations. Therefore, formal control of public health services has to be undertaken at a high level, creating the appropriate infrastructure and incentive systems within which organizations can work effectively and efficiently. Even where regulation is limited to these broader aims, focused at national rather than local issues, considerable expertise is required for it to be successful. Without appropriate understanding of the role of regulation and expertise in designing and implementing it, regulation can become burdensome, counterproductive and expensive and, at worst, ignored. The extent of compliance with regulation is frequently determined by the way in which it is implemented, which can also impact on the costs of compliance. Where costs are high, organizations and businesses are more likely to be prepared to risk non-compliance (National Audit Office 2000).

The lack of expertise in central government in understanding the role of regulation in the delivery of services has created too great a regulatory burden for services. In the NHS, much of the over-regulation has come from what have been called 'arms-length bodies'. These were national agencies, established to provide greater expertise in specific areas of service delivery. However, although knowledgeable about the specific areas for which they were responsible, they were not civil servants and, therefore, neither expert in regulation nor were they within the loop of the new drive by central government to improve regulation. The result was a proliferation of regulatory mechanisms, produced by each arms-length body, contributing to a vast array of often competing controls from central government. These concerns, plus others about over-regulation from elsewhere in the public sector, led to proposals to consider alternatives to regulation. It was felt that it had become too easy to write regulatory rules, without considering the control options open to central government departments. 'Regulation for its own sake is too often seen as an easy answer, without proper consideration being given to better ways of achieving the outcome' (Cabinet Office 1999 page 16).

Regulators

Governments tend to favour the establishment of regulatory bodies invested with statutory powers to prevent those public sector or private sector organizations that contribute to the fabric of public services organizations who persistently fail to comply with minimum standards from remaining in operation. Licencing of private sector operators particularly with regard to health care and care homes are common examples of this approach (see Table 5.1). Regulators are frequently but not always, independent of government departments. However, wherever located, they are intended to create controls that reflect a wider societal imperative. To enforce this, regulators are given sanctions to punish those who fail to comply with their requirements, in some cases through the power to prosecute (Public Audit Forum 2002 page 20).

Where governments have been at pains to avoid the full weight of creating an independent regulatory body, they face two choices in providing assurance to the public. They can either use monitoring processes conducted directly from central government departments or external reviews, which are frequently undertaken by independent bodies conducting a form of external

Table 5.1 Definitions of uses of assessment findings

Accreditation: A formal and voluntary process by which an independent body assesses and recognizes an organization as meeting or exceeding criteria. For example, accreditation by the Joint Commission is a determination that an eligible health care organization complies with applicable standards related to issues like patient safety.

Certification: The procedure and action by which the USA Department of Health and Human Services, Centers for Medicare and Medicaid Services (CMS) evaluates and recognizes (certifies) an institution that has met all requirements for participation in the Medicare program requirements or conditions.

Licensure: Authorization by law (usually at the state level) to perform the activities of a profession (such as medicine, dentistry, or nursing) or the operation of a facility (such as a hospital or ambulatory surgery center).

(Joint Commission on Accreditation of Healthcare Organisations http://www.jcaho.org/htba/ambulatory+care/surgical/deemed+status.htm#2)

review, using either inspection or audit. Both these approaches enable the imposition of externally-derived controls on organizations. Targets are used to set output levels which organizations have to demonstrate they have achieved. As pointed out earlier, in the public as in other sectors, performance targets provide information on past performance and not on whether the organization is focused on the right values and procedural justice. And as has been demonstrated in the case of health care, performance targets have tended to be a random selection of indicators, based on aspects of quality which have immediate political currency, and, therefore, generated by a central government department of health, which does not have a coherent view of the workings of the whole health care system. And not surprisingly, these sorts of performance measures can encourage what is called gaming, moving numbers around to present organizations in a better light than otherwise might be the case. This is frequently interpreted as misreporting and, occasionally, fraudulent reporting as demonstrated by the cases of misrepresentation of waiting list figures by a few hospital trusts.

> The British system of government has become excessively centralized over the past fifty years, and this has led to an increase in bureaucracy as Whitehall tries to ensure that its policies are being implemented effectively at local level. Separate systems for controlling spending and monitoring targets have proliferated, absorbing resources needed by teachers, doctors, police and social services.
>
> (Better regulation task force 2001)

Another approach is the creation of formal controls through criteria used in inspections or in accreditation systems. In this case, organizations are assessed for compliance with detailed criteria by external assessors working for an independent body or a government department or agency. The criteria can reflect either minimum standards that must be complied with, or more aspirational levels of service provision, which encourage the organizations to strive to achieve compliance.

The costs of scrutiny work are unknown but one study put a figure of £1billion per annum as the total direct costs of employing government inspectors, regulators, ombudsmen and statutory auditors. (Hood *et al.* 1999). This figure did not include compliance costs, which relate to the time staff in public bodies spend on activities linked to audit and inspection (Lord Sharman 2002 para 5.19). The study suggests such compliance costs are likely to dwarf the direct costs of the regulators themselves. External control in the provision of public services is a very expensive activity and while providing a degree of reassurance to the public and to politicians that their demands for processes are being met, does little to guarantee that public services really are improved (National Audit Office 2001b).

There will always be cases of people breaking laws and failing to meet mandatory requirements. In contrast, rules that have been developed very closely with, or indeed by, those whose behaviour is to be controlled might be more readily complied with. The rules should be targeted to ensure that they require the minimum standards necessary to deliver adequate protection. A common feature of all effective systems is that there is the potential for the imposition of real sanctions.

(Better regulation task force 2000a para 6.1)

Effective regulatory systems, in this interpretation, have rarely been directed at the quality of health care. In external review, particularly that based on standards, the definition of quality is enshrined within the standards and, therefore, determined by the inspectors. Governments rarely wish to be accused of bad management by independent external bodies, of the organizations they directly or indirectly own. In a system that is short of capacity, there is no scope for closure if an organization receives a poor inspection report. Removing organizations from the supply chain, while demand for health care is increasing would merely create more pressure on an already stressed system. Therefore, when the government has direct responsibility for the provision of services that are resource constrained, it is logical for there to be a preference for keeping monitoring and inspection within central government and to undertake this function from within the relevant government department. Departments wish to demonstrate that organizations are behaving according to the objectives and expectations of their political masters, but without being forced into declaring them as failing or unfit, which could result in the ultimate sanction of closing them down (Hood *et al.* 1998; Vass and Simmonds 2001a page 12).

Inspection tends to become a preferred option when there is a layer of government between the providers of services and central government, which can be held responsible for the quality of health care, or when health care is run by independent or private sector businesses. In this case, the controls are determined centrally and the power to require change through the imposition of sanctions or other pressures tends to also be held centrally. When regional governments, or more locally democratically accountable structures are introduced, it becomes possible for central government to support the idea of independent national inspection as a mechanism to hold local organizations to account to central government.

In addition, the principle of subsidiarity calls for power to be given to the administrative unit nearest to the citizen (Scott 2000). True devolution calls for both more open and localized demonstrations of accountability and this means that, for accountability to work, the power to call for change in deficient provider organizations must lie with the local community. Therefore, in a locally accountable system based on stakeholder involvement, the decisions about changes in actions and delivery must be controlled at the local level. In this case, it is possible to retain centralized inspection regimes and central performance management regimes to provide information for local bodies and stakeholders to judge services upon but not to recommend change. The judgements as to the satisfactoriness of organizational performance must lie with the local community.

Government control over the direct provision of services, therefore, spans a set of opportunities ranging from specification of good leadership and internal management systems, which is referred to as 'internal control', to the direct imposition of expected behaviours, which is referred to as 'external control'. Vass and Simmonds (2001a) point to a proliferation of reports emerging from both central government and local government. The foci of the documentation range from an evaluation of the role of leadership and risk management (internal control) in improving public service performance to the scrutiny of local government authorities responses to audit and inspection regimes (external control). The choice facing governments, therefore, lies in the extent to which systems will be encouraged to produce their own internal management systems or to be controlled by external systems. The latter approach is increasingly accepted as the way to ensure service quality as well as providing public accountability (Audit Commission 2003).

Therefore, the debate hinges on the difference between conformance with rules and regulation and performance in providing services effectively and efficiently. The recommendations for corporate governance, introduced into the private sector (Cadbury and The London Stock Exchange 1992; Hampel Committee report 1998; The Internal Control Working Party of the Institute of Chartered Accountants in England and Wales 1999) were influencing thinking in the public sector and government. When applied to government organizations and services, this view of corporate governance argued for 'lighter touch' external review and regulation (Vass and Simmonds 2001a), with review bodies working within a framework that expects service providers to implement good corporate governance procedures.

> Since these include verifiable (i.e. inspectable) internal controls for the management of risk and the establishment of performance targets, then the review bodies should expect the service providers themselves to have mechanisms to avoid poor outcomes and provide a framework of incentives and targets for achieving outcomes and being accountable for them. If so, lighter touch review and regulation is an inevitable outcome, and the cost-effective role of ongoing review becomes inspection of the systems of internal controls and procedures (a well established practice of external financial audit) to ensure they are sound and operating effectively. Action and

further 'heavier handed review' only occurs when they are found wanting.

(Vass and Simmonds 2001a page 6)

So, government was yielding to the persuasive arguments that assurance frameworks based on corporate governance principles could be used to provide the necessary guarantees that public services are providing care in an acceptable manner. But how, in this case, would the definition of acceptable be provided? The market-based arguments which supported the development of these ideas in the private sector were not available to the public sector – even where health care systems were being reformed to reflect market-based philosophies. Public expectations and public opinion on the way in which services are provided are believed to influence voting patterns. And the definition of quality in public services is provided from the views of the general public. The conclusion that was drawn was that public views are needed to provide the framework for the definition of quality of public services and then, correspondingly, they are needed to generate the framework for the provision of assurance to the public that services are provided as they require. But most importantly, the public can no longer be assumed to be willing to just accept what politicians and managers say. The current mood of public mistrust of public services requires independent assessment and verification for the public to know that it is being served appropriately. As Michael Power observed, increasing demands for accountability to different stakeholder constituencies generate a need for independent assessment and audit (Power 1997).

Stakeholders

'The New NHS Modern and Dependable' (CM 3807 1997), sets out the position and expectations concerning corporate governance in the NHS. The sixth principle is to 'Rebuild public confidence in the NHS as a public service accountable to patients, open to the public and shaped by their views.' There are many ways in which the public's views can be elicited and represented for accountability purposes. Should there be direct public consultation on how well organizations are doing? Or is this better done by consulting with other bodies who have a related interest in the service, for example, social services are affected by the local provision of health care? The solution that had emerged for the UK government had taken hold at the beginning of its first term of office. Public views could be incorporated based on what was then termed 'the stakeholder society' (Blair 1996).

However, defining stakeholders in public services is not an easy task. Public sector organizations tend to have multiple publics and multiple account-abilities. Stakeholder theory emerged, as shown above, to help with the definition of corporate governance in the private sector. An early view was that stakeholders included all affecters and affectees of corporate policies and activities (i.e. all relevant interests), which would include other organizations affected by any decisions taken (Friedman 1970). Historically, this definition was considered non-controversial and was widely applied. More recently, the argument has changed and stakeholder theory is based on a broadened theory of property rights, which demonstrates that all contributors to a firm's success have a legitimate moral claim to be beneficiaries of that success because they bear the risk of the activities carried out by the organization. One means of identifying stakeholders is through the actual or potential harms and benefits that they experience or anticipate experiencing as a result of the firm's actions or inactions (Friedman 1970).

Translating this idea into the public sector means that the consumers of services become the key stakeholders. Managers providing services to the public cause harm to the public if they fail to provide the expected services. Although other organizations may suffer as a consequence, and staff may be affected by changes in service provision, the key risk bearers are those people who suffer as a consequence of the poor provision of public services. This is most acute in situations where competition is limited. In these circumstances, the consumer voice becomes important. To develop what Hirschman (1970) describes as 'voice' 'within an organisation is synonymous with the history of democratic control through the articulation and aggregation of opinions and interests' (Hirschman 1970 page 55). In the case of health care, everyone is a potential patient. And therefore the wider public, who in effect own the services through the provision of taxes to fund them, have an interest in holding public services to account. However, this contradicts the logic of devolving management to local organizations, where it is claimed the purpose of local organizations is to serve a local community or public. Therefore, the population of a local area served by the public services are the key stakeholders. Government policy is not clear on this issue as there are two competing views of the local public served in the case of Foundation Hospitals. One is that the local community is of paramount importance, particularly for the protection of public health. The other is that Foundation Hospitals are free to treat whomsoever they choose and, therefore, their publics may be much wider than those living in the immediate locality.

More compelling, given the difficulty of defining which public groups should be included as stakeholders, is the argument that public services should consult on all decisions where uncertainty is high either because of the nature of the policies, or because of the difficulties in defining objectives and strategic risk. 'Experience shows that risk management decisions made in collaboration with stake-holders are more effective and more durable. Stakeholders are more likely to accept and implement a risk management decision they have participated in shaping' (The Presidential/Congressional Commission on Risk

Assessment and Risk Management 1997 page 16). Although this does not answer the question of how to define appropriately the public to be consulted, it does argue for the fact that public views must be incorporated into decision making as uncertainty cannot be handled scientifically or categorically. Uncertainty must, instead, be handled through judgement and negotiation. And this argues that the population or community to be included in the decision making must encompass those people who are directly affected by the risks taken by the organization.

> Stakeholder collaboration is particularly important for risk management because there are many conflicting interpretations about the nature and significance of risks. Collaboration provides opportunities to bridge gaps in understanding, language, values and perceptions. It facilitates an exchange of information and ideas that enables all parties to make informed decisions about reducing risks. Collaboration does not require consensus, but it does require that all parties listen to, consider and respect each other's opinions, ideas and contribution. (The Presidential/Congressional Commission on Risk Assessment and Risk Management 1997 page 17)

This presents an argument for ensuring that affected publics are consulted upon all risks that affect them. This would, therefore, encompass staff as well as patients and members of the public. It would also encompass policies to address local public health risks, as well as risks of failing to manage the local provision of services. But it also means that the key stakeholders must not only determine the significance of risks locally and determine the risk appetite of the organisation, they must also be the judges of how well the organization is being managed (that is, how well the organisation and its management are performing). 'Feedback is a pre-condition for self-regulation or self-governance' (Ashby 1968; Turnbull 1997). However, for stakeholders (whether they are staff or the local public using services) to have the will to act, they need a power base independent of management to protect them from being treated as whistle blowers. The stakeholders have to be given a legitimate role to comment on the performance of the management. And this then leads to a need to ensure appropriate and proper governance processes. If a firm is not to affect adversely its stakeholders through its actions or inactions, it requires governance processes that enable its stakeholders to participate in establishing standards for assessing performance (Donaldson and Preston 1995). This applies to all public sector organizations including local authorities.

> A common theme running through all of the Government's requirements is the need for local authorities to review the various systems and processes they have in place for managing both their own internal

affairs and their relationships with key stakeholders. Together, these systems and processes comprise corporate governance.

(CIPFA/SOLACE 2001 para 1.6)

It has, therefore, been assumed that more open decision making by organizations will provide stakeholders with the confidence and the assurance that decisions are being made satisfactorily on their behalf. 'The more open and honest organisations are with themselves about their performance, the more open and honest they can be with service users and the public. Better quality services are then more likely; improved performance and being more open will increase public trust' (Audit Commission 2003 page 9). This, in turn, requires that organizations are freer to relate to their own stakeholders, which requires good governance structures to underpin credibility and confidence. 'Being open through genuine consultation with stakeholders and providing access to full, accurate and clear information leads to effective and timely action and lends itself to necessary scrutiny' (CIPFA/SOLACE 2001 para 2.8).

But at what level should the independent assessment be exercised and should its scope and content be left to local determination? Government provision of services tends to assume there is virtue in national standardization of provision, to ensure equity in provision. This, it is argued, is achieved by consistent adherence to national standards which ensure every recipient of services has the same access to services across the country. In the past, it has been assumed that there should be a central control system, which will ensure that the standards are applied equally across the whole country. However, recently the arguments have changed. National standards have become instead the mechanism for ensuring the achievement of devolution. Instead, there should be local flexibility to interpret national standards, recognizing differences in local circumstances.

> The argument is sometimes advanced that national standards and devolution are incompatible, since the one represents centralized controls whereas the other should mean freedom from such accountability. However, demanding standards and devolution need to go together. The best way in which a national standard can be met is by recognising local and often individualized differences and giving service providers the flexibility to shape services around the needs and aspirations of customers and communities.
>
> (The Prime Minister's Office of Public Services Reform 2002 page 16)

This change in the interpretation of the application of national standards has arisen through growing awareness of what has been termed the complexity of the delivery chain. The distance from central government to the delivery systems of local services is often so great, with so many intermediate decision making bodies and service delivery organizations, that it is impossible to devise a single coherent system (National Audit Office 2004).

It is possible to set national standards and allow the development of local inspection and review. However, this could lead to the development of very different assessment tools and criteria at a local level, which give rise to post-code lotteries of service provision. Therefore, there are arguments for nationally agreed methods and tools for the conduct of inspection and review. But, to go full circle, external review or inspection competes with the growing ideology of corporate governance and internal leadership. External inspection tends to lead to over control, which stifles innovation and improved service development. The challenge for health care, therefore, is to find ways of achieving what has been termed a 'lighter touch' in terms of centralized inspection, encouraging local flexibility in management and service provision.

A number of different initiatives were introduced into the National Health Service to control its activities. Along with all the regulatory frameworks that existed to control all business, and those that were designed to control public service organizations, were those developed specifically to control the NHS. A national performance management framework was introduced to monitor the performance of the NHS. In addition, the Commission for Health Improvement was introduced as a national monitoring body. And thirdly, the internal control and risk management agenda was imposed on the NHS to correspond with the developments in central government.

The process of introducing internal controls in the NHS

Objectives as the focus for risk management began to gain significance, as they had in the governance of private businesses. Public Service Agreements were introduced as the stated objectives for government departments and for the services which were managed directly by departments. Public Service Agreements were designed to bring together in a single document the aim, objectives and performance targets of organizations into a single statement for each major service area, and should contain the following:

- Aim: a high-level statement of the role of the department.
- Objectives: in broad terms, what the department is looking to achieve.
- Performance targets: under most objectives, outcome-focused performance targets.
- Value for money: each department is required to have a target for improving the efficiency or value for money of a key element of its work.

- A statement of who is responsible for the delivery of these targets. Where targets are jointly held this is identified and accountability arrangements clearly specified.

Each government department was required to identify the risks to achieving these objectives. The Department of Health identified a wide range of risks covering the environment; consumer products; new technologies; terrorism; and medicines; as well as risks from behavioural lifestyles, such as smoking and drug and alcohol abuse; and also risks from adverse effects of medical and social care. However, as in other parts of government, public health risks tend not to be able to call upon formal, scientifically defended standards to the same extent as environment protection or occupational protection or occupational health and safety legislation. For public health, the focus for organizations is on how issues of risk are dealt with in general legislation and how much is left to individual organizations or individual members of the public to deal with. In the United States, for example, public health has tended to try to establish specific laws and regulatory mechanisms to address risks and make them a very visible and ideological component of public administration. In other administrations, such as those in the UK or in Australia, the preferred approach as been to create legislation which encourages and facilitates attention to questions of risk, rather than to impose regulation on organizations (Government of Victoria 2000).

By 2003 the Department of Health had recognized the need to bring together strategic risk and operational risk in a single process but was struggling to implement this. Strategic risks were to be set at a national level, in order to support the implementation of the Public Service Agreements, which stated the objectives for government departments. These are the top priority risks for the department identified under significant risk themes, currently: delivery of the Public Service Agreement; exercise of departmental statutory and other responsibilities; and organizational capability. The approach introduced was, therefore, adapted from the private sector approach to risk management. A strategic risk register was sought which would contain a variety of different risks. Some would relate to the achievement of strategic objectives as identified by the management board; some would have been escalated from programme/directorate/group risk registers which could not be managed at a lower management level and require a decision to be made by the board; and some would be external risks over which the Department of Health had no control but which required monitoring by the board so that contingency responses could be prepared. Service delivery, managed by independent bodies on behalf of the Department of Health, would have to provide assurances to the board that the risks were being appropriately managed.

In its approach, the Department of Health recognized two sorts of risks: those that are voluntarily taken, where its role might be restricted to providing the public with sufficient information to allow them to make their own choices; and involuntary risks – over which the individual has no control and where the public expects adequate safety provisions, such as those relating to wider or more serious public health concerns, or where vulnerable groups (like the poor or children) might be at risk. For these policy-related risks, the Department of Health had been attempting to follow central government guidance to make the risk management process more open and transparent, involving the public more fully, and improving the way risk is communicated to the public.

However, the NHS is organized to be a separate entity from state government and is structured to operate through boards, constituted to mimic the governance structures found in the private sector. The concerns of accountability here are with uncertainty of outcome of management action, rather than outcomes to which statistical probabilities can be assigned. These boards are encouraged to focus their attention on questions of risks, both public health and service delivery risks, within a corporate governance structure which was, during their emergence in the 1990s, based upon the recommendations created for private sector boards.

The growing recognition of the need for increased understanding of risk management, combined with the new formulation of corporate governance in the private sector, which emphasized internal controls based upon risk management, added fuel to the move to develop further corporate governance in the running of the NHS. As a consequence, a range of measures was introduced to provide a framework for corporate governance, which would incorporate internal control and risk management formally into the running of the NHS. In February 1995, Sir Alan Langlands, the then Chief Executive of the NHS, asked organizations whether they were able to sign a voluntary assurance statement on the effectiveness of their system of internal control as recommended in the 1992 Cadbury Committee report. In 1996, a system for improving internal controls within NHS organizations, called controls assurance, was introduced to bring all these measures together into a single initiative, which would establish a single coherent framework for the standardization of the approach to internal control across the National Health Service.

> All organisations require internal control but meet this requirement with different degrees of formality. However, there is general agreement that the greater the size of, and public interest in, an organisation, the more important it is for that organisation to establish and maintain a formal framework.
>
> (Department of Health 2001c page 2)

Controls assurance

Controls assurance was based on principles, established in order to demonstrate to the wider community that each board is 'not only satisfied that there is an integrated system to manage risk and improve healthcare but that such a system can be clearly described' (Department of Health 2001c page 2). Following on from the introduction of improved board structures and requirements for better governance, this was described as 'the final piece of the corporate governance jigsaw'.

Controls assurance was, therefore, created to bring together, in a single formalized and standardized model for the National Health Service, the principles enshrined in the Turnbull report, translated for use in government departments and then redefined for use by NHS board structures. It was also designed to reflect the recognized principles for internal control in government departments which were stated in many places, for example, the guidance for managers in governmental organizations (see table 5.2) Controls assurance was defined as:

> a holistic process designed to provide evidence that NHS bodies are doing their reasonable best to manage themselves so as to meet their objectives and protect patients, staff, the public and other stakeholders against risks of all kinds. Fundamental to the process is the effective involvement of people and functions within the organisation through application of self-assessment techniques.
>
> (NHS Executive 1999a page 2)

The key to the implementation of controls assurance was the introduction of an annual statement (a precursor to the statement on internal control) accompanying the annual report and annual accounts, which provides the general public with confirmation that the board of directors believes that these systems are in place and operating effectively. This enhanced the role of non-executive directors, placing them firmly in the driving seat of organizational development, making them responsible for the management of risks occurring from both the practices carried out within their organizations and the impact of external changes.

Although self-assessment underpinned the whole concept of assurance, it was recognized that there was a need to ensure that the statement covered appropriate areas and could be deemed what was termed 'fit for purpose' (NHS Executive 1998). It was decided that a verification process should be introduced to review evidence that the risk management strategy had been produced and that it was being regularly reviewed and updated, and that appropriate actions and improvements would be introduced where lack of control had been identified.

Table 5.2   Framework for establishing and maintaining effective internal control
Adapted from International Organisation of Supreme Audit Institutions

---

Managers' internal control roles and responsibilities
- Create a positive control environment by providing:
  - a positive ethical tone
  - guidance for proper behaviour
  - a lack of temptations for unethical behaviour
  - discipline when appropriate
  - a written code of conduct for employees.
- Ensure that personnel have and maintain a level of competence to perform their duties.
- Clearly define key areas of authority and responsibility.
- Establish clear lines of reporting.
- Establish management control policies and procedures that are based on management's analysis of risk.
- Reinforce the importance of management control.
- Monitor the organization's control operations through annual assessment and reports to top management.

Common internal control practices
- Internal control practices are often designed to comply with internal control standards developed and promulgated by a central authority.
- The workforce is effectively trained and managed so as to achieve results.
- Performance indicators are developed and monitored.
- Key duties and responsibilities are divided among people to reduce the risk of error and fraud.
- Managers compare actual performance to planned or expected results.
- Information processing is controlled through checks on data.
- Physical controls safeguard assets.
- Access to resources is limited to authorized individuals.
- Transactions are authorized and carried out only by authorized persons.
- Transactions are recorded.
- Internal control is clearly documented.

Controls assurance also developed at a time when there was a desire to develop what was called 'single audit', which describes an approach to unifying audit in order to avoid the burden of over-audit, characterized by uncoordinated, overlapping controls and audits. The single audit approach required 'the development of an integrated internal control structure in which checks carried out at higher levels in the system rely in part on checks carried out at lower levels' (Caldeira 2000 page 2). For this to occur, it was necessary to establish a common controls framework, with a minimum set of control and audit standards. It also went hand in hand with the aspiration of having the requisite decentralized management: 'in principle, meet ex ante minimum standards of internal control . . . with the objective of ensuring sound functioning of the control systems and the legality/regularity of operations. There must be acceptance of full disclosure by management. Through the system there will need to be assurance statements submitted by the different organisations involved' (Caldeira 2000 page 3).

NHS organizations were advised to adopt a top-down, risk-profiling exercise to assess the management of risk, thereby enabling organizations to 'take stock of existing strengths and weaknesses, focus upon overlaps and gaps in control, as well as helping to identify and rank the key risks they need to monitor and measure' (NHS Executive 1998). It was acknowledged that these processes need to be driven from the top of the organization and that the Chief Executive, as accountable officer, should establish a sub-committee of the board to oversee the process. It was also recommended that all directors should have an opportunity to contribute to the top-down, risk-profiling exercise. Once this was complete, other groups of staff could be involved more extensively in risk assessment and risk management, enabling consolidation, rationalization and completion of the control framework (NHS Executive 1998).

The introduction of the original controls assurance statement was phased over a three-year period of time. In 1997/8, boards of directors were required to produce a statement on internal financial control. By 1999, the consolidated accounts for the NHS carried a statement of assurance on the system of internal control across all NHS financial systems. But the ambition was to produce a consolidated statement that covered the whole of the system of internal control for the NHS. In short, this would hold the Chief Accounting Officer for the NHS (the Chief Executive) accountable for all the management of all parts of the NHS including clinical services (NHS Executive 1998). This would be achieved by consolidating all the statements on internal control from all the individual NHS organizations into one overall statement for the NHS as a whole.

The name controls assurance suggests that its purpose is to provide assurance on the system of internal control and (linked inextricably, as in the governance literature) the control of risk. The effectiveness of controls could only be assessed, and assurance given, by examining whether risks existed. Identification and assessment of specific risks in health care organizations, it was argued, required highly-specialized knowledge. Therefore, the specialists (that is, those people who provide the services) had to undertake risk assessment in their own areas and to report on their satisfaction with how these risks were being managed. The increasing specialization in all jobs, but in health care in particular, means that managers are less able to closely supervise their subordinates. How then can the individual know the 'rules' under which they are to work (Morley 2004)? The board's assurance derives from the system in place, in which staff are happy with the level of risks they face. The board, therefore, needs to know first, that the staff have undertaken the task and second, that they are not facing any unacceptable risks. As the board is not expert enough to assess all risks, it has to devise a system which can report to them that all the activities taking place in the organization are being as well conducted as they can reasonably be. Furthermore, there was a growing interest in how to improve quality in health care and the need to introduce continuous quality improvement. If quality improvement is the aspiration, then risks to improving quality must be assessed and assurance given that the internal controls on the quality improvement system are effective.

Controls assurance standards

In 1999, a new circular was introduced which explained further the requirements set out the previous year and described the controls for non-clinical areas as wider organizational controls. 'At a time when many other management challenges face NHS organisations, one of the key objectives of the controls assurance is to ensure that the task is made less onerous through the development of a comprehensive "control framework"' (NHS Executive 1999a para 7). As with all developments in internal control there was a need to set internal control standards, developed and promulgated by a central authority, in this case the Department of Health (International Organisation of Supreme Audit Institutions 2001). Along with this circular, 18 risk management and organizational control standards were issued covering topics which were considered to pose significant operational risks to NHS organisations (see table 5.3). A further organization standard on research governance was issued in 2003.

The standards were designed to cover significant organizational risk areas and pull together into one place the large number of relevant existing laws and NHS Executive circulars which impact on the delivery of services in the NHS. To conform with the accepted views on internal control, such as those from COSO and CoCo, that a model of internal control should underpin management and audit activity in this area, a model was drawn up to reflect the understanding of management and internal control in the NHS. This reflected the agreed principles for internal control, particularly emphasizing the importance of clear lines of accountability and defined roles and responsibilities; clear processes and risk management; competent staff; and adequate performance indicators to assess internal control (International Organisation of Supreme Audit Institutions 2001). The standards were then framed around the model of internal control and the criteria were 'drawn from current statutory and mandatory requirements together with relevant best practice guidance. The aim is to integrate the many and varied existing requirements within a common framework' (NHS Executive 1999a para 8) (see figure 5.1).

In the introduction to the circular, Sir Alan Langlands explained that in future years, the self-assessment against the standards would form the basis of

Table 5.3 Controls assurance standards
Buildings, land and plant
Catering
Decontamination of medical devices
Environmental management
Fire safety
Fleet and transport
Health and safety
Human resources
Infection control
Information management and technology
Medical devices management
Medicines management
Professional advice
Purchasing and supply
Research management
Security
Waste management

Core standards
Governance
Risk management
Financial management

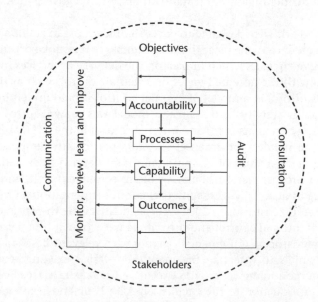

Figure 5.1 Internal control model for the NHS.

a consolidated assurance statement covering all risks and risk management set out in 'one clear, comprehensive and cohesive structure' (NHS Executive 1999a). In the first year of the standards, NHS organizations were asked to conduct a baseline self-assessment of compliance with the risk management and organizational control standards and to formulate a prioritized action plan with clearly assigned responsibilities (NHS Executive 1999a).

During 1998 it became clear that the introduction of the statement on internal control was an ambitious requirement for NHS organizations (NHS Executive 1998). Health service organizations were struggling to cope with the additional assurance statement. They were not alone in this, surveys of the commercial sector were showing that firms were experiencing similar problems (Deloitte and Touche 2000). It was recognized at this time that there were complex issues in extending governance and assurance relating to clinical areas. At this time an additional concept, known as clinical governance, was also introduced into the governance agenda for NHS organizations. Clinical governance emerged as a concept in 1998, intended to provide NHS organizations and individual health care professionals with a framework on which to build a single coherent, local programme for quality improvement (NHS Executive 1999b). From April 1999, all English hospital Chief Executives were given a statutory responsibility for the quality of patient care, which requires them to keep a firm eye on how well surgeons, doctors, nurses and support staff do their jobs. They have to ensure that doctors who are identified as performing poorly either retrain, change their caseloads or leave their jobs. Clinical governance aimed at preventing the types of incident, crises or serious failures that are significant because they represent a failure to deliver a safe and effective service. In addition, it set out a series of clinical quality standards, with mechanisms for local delivery of high quality clinical services, together with a monitoring programme for ensuring safety and efficiency (Department of Health 2002c para 1.20).

Clinical governance

In 1998, the NHS Executive decided, in anticipation of the introduction of the concept of clinical governance, to bifurcate the assurance statement into two separate elements: non-clinical and clinical assurances, with clinical quality covered in a separate annual report on quality. 'The statement is intended to provide an overall assurance that the organisation has a comprehensive risk management strategy in place to cover all significant non-clinical areas. It is anticipated that clinical governance issues will be reported upon separately through the annual quality report' (NHS Executive 1998). Clinical risk was, therefore, deliberately separated from non-clinical risk. Because of this, the orthodoxy of risk management approaches of assessment and using tools, such as risk registers and risk matrices, and controls in the forms of action plans and risk prioritization were applied only to non-clinical risk. From 1999/2000, every NHS organization was required to have a strategy for dealing with non-clinical risk only (NHS Executive 1998).

Clinical governance provided a framework within which local organizations could work to improve and assure the quality of clinical services for patients. It also set out a series of clinical quality standards, with mechanisms for local delivery of high quality clinical services, together with a monitoring programme for ensuring safety and efficiency (Department of Health 2002c para 1.20). Clinical governance defined the values, the culture, the processes and the procedures that must be put in place in order to achieve sustained 'quality of care' both within and between the organizations that make up the NHS (see table 5.4).

> Clinical governance can be defined as a framework through which NHS organisations are accountable for continuously improving the quality of their services and safeguarding high standards of care by creating an environment in which excellence in clinical care will flourish . . . Clinical governance involves above all shifting the level of quality provided by the majority of health organisations – those in the middle range of performance – closer to the exemplars services in the NHS.
>
> (NHS Executive 1999b page 6)

Clinical governance is primarily concerned with quality and is built upon assumptions of continuous quality improvement, while recognizing the need to ensure safety of patient care (Scally and Donaldson 1998). However, the board of health care organizations had to develop a mechanism for assessing not only its formal internal control, that is its recognized procedures and processes (a mechanism provided by controls assurance), but also a mechanism to assess its clan or informal internal controls.

The theory of internal control as pronounced by Turnbull, based upon the understanding of all organizational risks, is difficult to implement in

Table 5.4 Main components of clinical governance

Clear lines of responsibility and accountability for the overall quality of clinical care.

A comprehensive programme of quality improvement activities.

Clear policies aimed at managing risk including controls assurance which promote self-assessment to identity and manage risks and clinical risk systematically assessed with programmes in place to reduce risk.

Procedures for all professional groups to identify and remedy poor performance.

---

health care organizations that are extremely complex and multi-faceted. Health care generates a large number of risks and boards struggle to deal with the whole range. They cannot monitor the actions of every doctor and other professional who, by the very nature of medicine, deals continuously with risks and potential harm to patients. Board assurance in this area can only operate at the level of trust in professional staff, ensuring they are appropriately trained and competent for the work they undertake and subscribe to appropriate professional values, which recognize the changing expectations of patients and the public. Clinical governance is, therefore, a control system specifically designed to enable boards to tackle assurance of those informal or clan internal controls used to control and change professional behaviour and activity.

Controls assurance and clinical governance had evolved separately but were originally felt to be linked through a shared focus on risk management. 'Controls assurance and clinical governance go hand-in-hand linked principally through risk management processes. Clinical governance provides assurances on the mechanisms (or controls) in place to improve the quality of clinical care and manage clinical risk' (Controls Assurance Team 1999 para 14), whereas an effective risk management system combined with organizational controls would provide a 'solid foundation upon which to build an environment in which quality care can be provided and clinical excellence can flourish . . . "getting the organisation right" will significantly increase the likelihood of achieving the desired outcomes in relation to meeting the needs of patients.' (Controls Assurance Team 1999).

Creating standards for risk management

Despite the initial separation of controls assurance and clinical governance, it was suggested that there was potential for adopting a holistic (integrated) approach to risk management, encompassing both clinical and non-clinical aspects through extending the control framework to include standards for clinical risk management. The single set of clinical standards would be produced by the controls assurance team, the NHS Litigation Authority and other key stakeholders within the Department of Health working together. The first step would be to refine the standards in the NHS Litigation Authority's clinical negligence scheme for Trusts (CNST) (used to determine the insurance premiums to be paid by NHS organizations), in order to produce a basis for the future development of clinical risk management standards (Controls Assurance Team 1999). It was also intended that there would also be a common set of standards which would cover recording, reporting, investigation and analysis of incidents, complaints and claims across clinical and non-clinical areas in line with the Chief Medical Officer's report, 'Learning from experience' (Controls Assurance Team 1999). Organization-wide risk management would also produce the desired risk register and the ability to prioritize the portfolio of risks being managed by NHS organizations, in particular NHS Trusts.

The approach to risk was to be positive and strategic, rather than just focusing on the reduction of risks associated with hazards. The Australian and New Zealand definition of risk management was accepted as underpinning these developments in which risk management is defined as 'the culture, processes and structures that are directed towards the effective management of potential opportunities and adverse effects' (Standards Australia 1999 page 4).

In 2001, the original eighteen standards, which included a general risk management system standard, had been supplemented by two new standards for governance and for financial management – making a total of twenty. Each standard continued to contain criteria which followed a model for internal control (Controls Assurance Team 1999). Controls assurance was described as developing into a fully comprehensive health care management process (Reeves 2000). It was seen at this time as more than just a process encompassing non-clinical risk management based on organizational standards but was intended to become the whole process underpinning the governance arrangements for the NHS, including financial governance, non-clinical governance and clinical governance. A new governance standard, introduced to be an over-arching standard to assist boards in their strategic approach to the management of internal control, set the control criteria at board level for all three elements: financial; organizational (non-clinical); and clinical control. Boards would be able to judge their activities against these standards and sign off a comprehensive assurance statement which would assure patients, staff, the public, politicians and, most importantly, the Chief Executive of the NHS that all boards were doing their reasonable best to manage risks of all kinds and, in so doing, afford protection to patients, staff and other stakeholders. This new standard, combined with the organization-wide risk management standard would provide the bed-rock for the whole of the controls assurance process, helping boards to systematically review risk across their organizations and addressing the need for an overall system of internal control. The remainder of the standards would provide the necessary information for assurances on risks associated with specific areas of the management of the business of health care organizations.

The introduction of the single governance standard was a major shift in the emphasis of controls assurance towards a 'comprehensive health care management process'. It heralded a move away from the dominance of the organizational standards towards the development of a management paradigm intended to improve the quality of health care. The final piece of the jigsaw – the shift towards a single model for promoting corporate governance in dealing with uncertainty in management decisions – had been slotted into place. The key to implementing this lay in the development of the comprehensive assurance statements required by the maturity model, which laid out the process of internal control expected of NHS organizations that had evolved over the development of controls assurance.

External verification continued to be recognized as important. The concept of the single audit against a single internal control model, however, had disappeared. The introduction of the Commission for Health Improvement provided an extra player in the assessment process along with the Audit Commission and other audit bodies, such as the Health and Safety Executive, the Medical Devices Agency and the Medicines Controls Agency. It was decided that instead of continuing with the development of the single control model, to attempt to identify an 'optimum external verification methodology'.

In February 2001, the system of internal control took a step further towards a standardized approach to organization-wide risk management. In a letter from the Director of Finance, the single term 'governance' was used, pulling together for the first time the two concepts of corporate governance and clinical governance. Under the heading, governance convergence, it was stated that the Department of Health was 'committed to achieving a fully integrated approach to governance where clinical and corporate governance sit side by side – clinical governance focusing on continuous improvements in quality and corporate governance focusing on continuous improvements on having the necessary systems in place to minimize risk' (Reeves 2001). By 2005 it was intended that, under the single, internal control system, described as controls assurance, there would be fully-operational clinical risk management systems in place and working effectively. These systems would be based on controls assurance standards incorporating the NHS Litigation Authority's clinical risk management standards and supported by the recommendations coming out of National Institute for Clinical Excellence, which evaluated evidence for clinical practice and the National Service Frameworks.

But, by May 2001, the holistic approach to integrated governance and risk management had changed direction. Instead, a distinction was drawn between different forms of assurance: clinical assurance; organizational assurance; and financial assurance. These would come from different sources: the clinical governance annual report; the annual report; and the annual accounts, respectively. Boards would have to gain assurance by drawing on the wide variety of review processes that existed covering internal audit, health and safety, risk management, quality assurance, clinical audit and so on. The change in direction was due, in part, to a new requirement, issued for implementation in the following year from HM Treasury, which changed the Statement on Internal Control to align it with the Turnbull guidance on internal control. All centrally-funded organizations would be required to sign a full, as opposed to a partial, statement of internal control by the end of 2003.

Scoring against the standards

Based upon standards that codified the legal and other central requirements, organizations were allowed to assess their own risks and to decide the extent to which they were doing their reasonable best by scoring the standards. In theory, an organization doing what it perceived to be a good job in the light of difficult circumstances could give itself a high score, even though it may not be complying with all the requirements. Equally, organizations could be content with a low score, if this was felt to reflect their reasonable best in the circumstances in which they found themselves. These scores could not, therefore, be taken as indications of simple compliance with legislation. They were to be seen as indicators of levels of managed risk. The important information is not the score but the distance from a 100 per cent score. An organization with a high score might still experience catastrophic failure but this would be due to events beyond the control of the board and the organization. This process of assessing against the standards was to be subject to verification. Action plans would be submitted to demonstrate that organizations were doing their reasonable best to improve their situation. There was much talk of prioritization and how this should be achieved by organizations. Tools were discussed which would aid with this process. The difficulty that arose was that these tools were very helpful in determining capital expenditure, but they were less useful in making decisions about management processes.

However, the interpretation of the scoring of the standards shifted, almost on their release, to one of compliance rather than risk. Rather than being self-assessment tools for organizations to use to provide assurance on significant risks, the standards were seen as inspection tools. This was understandable as the standards were created around compliance requirements placed upon the NHS and the messages contained in the COSO system, which were influencing the interpretation of controls assurance by auditors, and emphasized the need to ensure compliance with existing laws and regulations. The re-interpretation of controls assurance by auditors created the unintended consequence of what has become recognized as the conundrum at the centre of controls assurance. If legislation exists, it must be complied with, but NHS organizations did not have the resources to comply with everything at once. Therefore, they were encouraged to prioritize their actions and related expenditure, and must, by definition, be content to live with certain levels of risk. However, it was not possible for the Department of Health to give permission to organizations to not comply with the law. Compliance competed with assurance in an unexpected way.

To add the provision of assurance against the standardized approach to the assessment of control systems, a list of examples of verification was included in each standard. Boards were expected to provide evidence they had done their reasonable best to develop control systems to manage the risks addressed by the standards. Although never intended to be the verification criteria for proving the existence of the control system, but merely an indication of things a board might like to take into account, many organizations and their auditors interpreted these as checklists of compliance against the standard. The net result was different perceptions of the role of the standardized system of internal control across the NHS, with some viewing it as an assessment of risk and others perceiving that verification examples were, in fact, checklists to be ticked. Some auditors produced algorithms to determine the precise level of compliance. The focus on compliance also raised questions about the validity of using scoring approaches to provide assurance at a national level. The central collection of the scores, originally intended merely to encourage organizations to carry out the assessment process, was reinterpreted both within the NHS and in some parts of the Department of Health as a measure of compliance. Research conducted into the scoring has demonstrated that, although there is statistical consistency in the way in which the scores are generated internally within an organization, enabling the board to compare scores for assurance purposes, the scoring patterns are not consistent from one organization to another (Wilde, Jones and Scrivens 2004). This means that although the scores can be used for the purposes of internal board assessment, they should not be used for external performance management. However, the central collection of data encouraged some parts of the Department of Health and some of its agencies to try to use the scores for performance management purposes. The result was a reification of the scores, in which internal guesses at scores, suitable only for internal management purposes, became believed to contain some legitimate form of measurement.

The objective of controls assurance was to produce a single, coherent system for developing controls against risks across the NHS, ultimately providing assurance at all levels that the NHS is being managed in line with developing expectations of public accountability. The project began by identifying specific risk areas for the NHS, which could impact on their objective of minimizing risks to patients during health care treatment. The process aided the identification of risk and the associated controls. However, the controls were intended to be open to local interpretation – there being no single management solution to managing a particular risk. Boards were asked to say they had, in the light of their local domestic agenda, done their reasonable best to deal with the management of the risks they faced, which included compliance with legislation and regulations. Health care around the world is subject to considerable regulation to ensure its safe provision. And for this reason, there is a always a tension between the desire of central authorities to control health care and the desire to permit local discretion in the provision of services. The definition of reasonable board behaviour and reasonable assurance is difficult and open to different interpretations.

At the beginning of 2003, the assurance agenda for the NHS was beginning to take shape. Clinical governance had begun to take root in the NHS and was propounding a philosophy of patient-centred care based on expressed values of humanity, equity, justice and respect, and emphasizing the centrality of the patient experience to health care. The term governance was being used to describe the overall system of accountabilities and assurances that must be put into place within an organization to ensure that it discharges its functions legally, effectively and ethically. There was a return to the distinction between corporate and clinical governance in which boards were exhorted to 'strike an appropriate balance between attention to the broader fiscal and corporate responsibilities encompassed by "corporate governance" and to the specific safety, quality and transformation agendas and issues encompassed by "clinical governance"' (Clinical governance support team and the national primary and care trust development programme 2003 section 3 page 2).

Boards had to be able to provide assurance on all risks and all controls and, therefore, rapidly had to find a way of describing systems that covered their whole organization. The Department of Health issued guidance to help boards develop a new, integrated approach to assurance in what was termed 'the assurance framework' (Department of Health 2002a page 3). In order to demonstrate the achievement of this goal, and to be able to sign the Statement on Internal Control, boards were required to document their assurance framework, where this is defined as: 'An assurance framework must be driven by the objectives of the organisation. In turn, the principal risks that might prevent those objectives being met need to be clear. This necessitates the existence of an embedded risk management culture and process throughout the organisation' (Department of Health 2002a page 3).

The challenge facing NHS boards to fulfil their responsibilities cannot be underestimated. Boards are required to have a sound understanding of the principal risks facing their organizations and they need to determine the level of assurance that should be available to them with regard to those risks.

> The difficulty is that there are many individuals, functions and processes within and outside an organisation that produce assurances. These range across statutory functions such as health and safety; to regulatory inspections that may or may not be NHS-specific; to voluntary accreditation schemes; and to management and other employee assurances. Taking stock, at any one point in time, of all these activities and their connection, or not, to key risks is a substantial but necessary task.
>
> (Department of Health 2002a page 3)

On 18 September 2003, new wording for the Statement on Internal Control for inclusion in the 2003/04 annual accounts (designed to bring the NHS fully in line with HM Treasury requirements) was published by the Department of Health. The key changes included: a requirement for accountable officers to identify how the risk management processes are maintained and developed to ensure continuing effectiveness; a requirement for disclosure of significant internal control issues; a requirement for a description of the processes in place at the organization; a requirement for documented evidence of the assessment of the effectiveness of the system of internal control and assurances that actions are or will be taken where appropriate to address issues arising. There would be no provision for partial statements for 2003/04 and beyond.

The preparation of assurance frameworks was suggested to be the appropriate method for achieving compliance with the Statement on Internal Control. The guidance stated that an assurance framework must be driven by the objectives of the organization. 'In turn, the principal risks that might prevent those objectives need to be clear which necessitates the existence of an embedded risk management culture and process throughout the organisation' (Department of Health 2002a page 4). It was suggested that:

> A common starting point is a structured risk identification and assessment exercise involving Board members and senior managers. Wider exercises with front line staff can be conducted subsequently. The aim is to define and generate a more detailed understanding of the organisation's objectives as well as a consensus over principal risks. This can then be viewed alongside subsequent analysis of existing and potential control and assurance sources.
>
> (Department of Health 2002a Page 4)

The guidance also recommended the establishment of a multidisciplinary assurance team with wide-ranging senior representation, which would help develop the assurance framework and would begin the process of integrating what was called 'health-care governance' across the organization, thus reintroducing the idea of an organization-wide risk management and control system.

The impact of controls assurance

Controls assurance was an attempt to provide a standardized approach to organization-wide risk management, internal control and assurance across the many different organizations that work in the NHS. When introduced, it was in advance of almost any other governance model that combined internal control and organization-wide risk management. Controls assurance was an ambitious project for the Department of Health, aimed at developing an

NHS-wide integrated risk and control system so sought after in the private sector, as described in Chapter 3, and toyed with by central government, as described in Chapter 4. It was elegant in the simplicity of the approach, which covered not only individual organizations but through summing them all together, would provide an assurance for the NHS as a whole. However, it existed alongside another control system, clinical governance, which was designed to deal with the vitally important professional clan controls, and also alongside other inspection and performance measurement systems. Taken together these multiple systems created complexity, over-control and could not be interpreted by managers, the Department of Health and auditors alike as an independent flexible management system, which could deliver the devolved management agenda. In the desire to generate assurance, the Department of Health had lost sight of the need to ensure that controls are not more onerous than the risks they seek to control. They had also forgotten the vision of the single audit, upon which the theory of internal control is based, which is aimed to reduce the amount of external assessment and direct central control. The regulatory instinct of the Department of Health had overtaken the virtues of the principles of an integrated risk management and control system designed to promote board autonomy.

The moves towards a single integrated approach to assurance into which controls assurance, clinical governance and the other governances were merging was a positive attempt to reintroduce the approach, to single audit. In its structure and approach, the single assurance approach contained within controls assurance had many similarities with the model of stakeholder management prescribed in the book entitled 'The Stakeholder Corporation', the approach adopted by the Labour party when it was first elected in 1997.

> The organisation takes full responsibility for managing its own performance according to documented procedures and criteria; the organisation also embraces communication feedback loops to enable it to learn from successes and failures in order to improve performance. Both the management system and the delivered performance are subject to periodic external accreditation or verification by a third party assessor.
>
> (Wheeler and Silanpaa 1997 page 164)

However, although accepting the methodology outlined, the NHS did not go the whole way in adopting the stakeholder approach when developing its approach to control and risk management. The controls assurance model and the later assurance framework followed the recommendations for health and safety risk management, and the model for providing assurance on controls. But the stakeholder approach recommended that companies should have professional units of stakeholder accounting and auditing, which need to be operationally independent but report direct to the company leadership. 'They should embrace an appropriate array of professional disciplines and should aim their reports at those operational areas of the company which maintain direct relationships with stakeholders' (Wheeler and Silanpaa 1997 page 166). Controls assurance did recognize the need to have professional involvement in the identification of risks and the need for independent verification provided by internal audit. The further development of the assurance framework extended the concerns of boards to organization-wide risk management focused on objectives. But in a health care system which was emphasizing decentralization of decision making another element would be needed, that is, the direct involvement of stakeholders in the definition of strategic risks, which would provide the needed link to supply a stakeholder assessment of performance.

It has been argued that stakeholder involvement is necessary for true accountability to be delivered. The regular process of auditors reporting the findings of their investigations to a local audit committee rather than reinforcing the independence of the auditor, tend to bond the auditor to the audit committee rather than to the stakeholders (Turnbull 2003). The introduction of local authority scrutiny of health care organizations perhaps provides the opportunity for this to develop (Audit Commission 2001).

The NHS Plan introduced scrutiny to reinforce local authorities' role in the leadership of the community and the promotion of local health. The role of the scrutiny committees is to provide independent (non-politically-partisan) monitoring of health service activities and plans. It is intended that these committees will select scrutiny topics concerning the development of local services. A truly decentralized model would require stakeholders to be fully involved in the setting of objectives for health care organizations and could review the effectiveness of internal controls with advice from the internal auditor, thus ensuring appropriate governance and accountability for health care organizations. The governance structures of Foundation Trusts are very much closer to this model of stakeholder involvement in the management of NHS organizations.

Chapter summary

This chapter has dealt with the following points:

- How the drive to devolve power to NHS organizations has led to an increase in review and regulatory bodies to monitor these devolved organizations.
- The types of controls needed to create successful regulation.
- The role of stakeholders in creating controls systems.
- The process of introducing internal controls in the NHS from setting objectives, to creating controls assurance and controls assurance standards, to introducing the concept of clinical governance, to combining controls assurance and clinical governance in a single standard for risk management.
- The use of standards as a scoring mechanism.
- The impact of controls assurance.

6 The Case for Change

Governments no longer find it necessary to create public value by direct service delivery. Instead it is argued, governments can add value by focusing on improving the quality of their decision making for policy and improving the achievement of outcomes. The main source of public value is 'trust, legitimacy and confidence. Trust is at the heart of the relationship between citizens and government. It is particularly important in relation to services which influence life and liberty – health and policing. If formal service and outcome targets are not met, a failure of trust will effectively destroy public value' (Strategy unit 2002 page 17). How then, in a world where governments are trying to let go of direct control of health care organizations to allow local management of services and encourage local innovation in service delivery and design, can the government ensure a national and equitable health service? How can health services be held to account for the provision of quality of health care that is guaranteed to all citizens? The preceding chapters have examined the options available to a government wishing to control the quality of health care, while at the same time conforming to the emerging model of new governance that encourages autonomy in devolved organizations. The solution has to lie in the construction of a form of governance and assurance that enables organizations to demonstrate how well they are making decisions, rather than central government prescribing the decisions for them.

The UK government has tended in the past to seek organizational structures which create an accountable hierarchy of organizations, in order to facilitate direct control of the delivery system. But this is no longer appropriate for a health care system in which public services are provided increasingly by private organizations at a time when the bureaucratic basis for trust in public services has eroded (Garsten and Grey 2001). The introduction of Foundation Trusts, which will be run and overseen by local stakeholders, patients, staff, local voluntary organizations and local authorities as board members, necessitates a new look at control. Foundation Trusts are based on a broader model of stakeholder involvement. The conundrum facing any government in determining the appropriate role for itself in regulation, is that where there is a broad range of stakeholders with varying interests (such as in the case of GPs) the state cannot take on its traditional objective role.

> Where there is a range of interests (some overlapping and some conflicting) it is not possible for the state to step in to balance two polarized positions. Both the state and the public have a collective interest as well as potentially an interest in individual cases. This is complicated further when, as in the case of GPs, the state is responsible (as employer or contractor) for the provision of services to the public. Therefore balancing the interests of service provider and service recipient is not a role that the state can easily play as an external, third party.
>
> (Better regulation task force 2000a para 5.1.2)

Devolved management

Assurance is required but is not easy to produce in a system as complex as the NHS, particularly when power is being devolved from the centre. Devolution of power to organizations has not been subject to extensive analysis as yet, but there are lessons learnt from the devolution of governmental power across the UK that raise issues which are likely to be similar for considerations of governance within the context of devolved power in the NHS. Devolution, it has been claimed, is the most radical constitutional reform seen in Britain since the Great Reform Act of 1832 because it seeks to reconcile two apparently conflicting principles: the sovereignty or supremacy of Parliament and the granting of self-government in domestic affairs (Bogdanor 1998). The issues arising from the devolution of national governance, as experienced in the cases of Scotland and Wales, present similar issues to those arising for local public service organizations obtaining new powers.

The devolution of governmental responsibility to health care organizations, as with other decision-making bodies, will create multilevel governance, with a variety of sovereignties involving multiple agencies with shared and overlapping constitutional authorities (Scott 2000). Devolution enshrines the principle of subsidiarity, which is that the competence for a policy should be given to the level of governance that can discharge it most effectively and this should be as close to the citizen as possible. In order for this to happen democratically, subsidiarity requires that citizens have a constitutional voice to affect local policies. But as Scott (2000) comments, experience of the devolution of power to regional governments across Europe has demonstrated that 'a pervasive feature of the organization of the contemporary global economy is the emergence of international institutions which incorporate binding and enforceable rules and which are replacing the organizations of (commercial) diplomacy hitherto based on voluntary codes, behavioral norms, and policy discretion' (Scott 2000 page 20). The same issue is replicated for the NHS in which decision making is devolved to local organizations. There will be pressure arising from the need to retain some element of standardization for purposes of equity and fairness in treatment, which will require, in turn, greater formalization of the definition of quality while at the same time creating localized governance structures that retain the freedom of local organizations to have power of their own decision making.

In addition, there are two other issues that are pertinent to governance which arise when devolution is implemented: policy overlap and policy contagion. Policy overlap occurs when two independent tiers of government have the ability to create the same policy, and can be dealt with either by restricting the powers of the devolved body or by requiring consultation on specific matters. Policy contagion occurs when one devolved body makes decisions that impact upon another devolved body. Both these are equally likely to be problems for devolved health care organizations, which result from the move from a singular to a pluralist (or multilevel) governance system. It will be necessary to change the culture and the behaviour of the civil service who generate central controls, if new governance for health services is to succeed.

> To borrow a metaphor, the civil service can be characterized as the 'software' of the 'operating system' that is British governance, without which the operating system will not function . . . Devolution has changed the internal configuration of the operating system of British governance; it has changed the structure of governance from singular to pluralist. Accordingly, the software that drives the operating system must be 'up-graded' to ensure that the re-configured system can execute efficiently the extended range of tasks now required of it, and be able to resolve unanticipated problems that may arise.
>
> (Scott 2000 page 11)

A new civil service culture to deliver new regulatory approaches for the NHS is required, which will encourage the separation of government responsibility for overall policy from the regulation function by identifying failures on behalf of the providers, in terms of service provision and also in the market in which they operate (Vass and Simmonds 2001a).

Alternative forms of regulation

The traditional approach to regulation, within which sanctions are applied to the enforcement of minimum standards, had been found to be inadequate.

This form of regulation could not cover all the public requirements for assurance that everything being done in the public's name is acceptable (Better regulation task force 2000a, 2000b). There are alternatives to this form of regulation covering a continuum of approaches ranging from self-regulation (or alternatives to state regulation) where there is no government involvement, right across to those schemes that are created and managed by government but stop short of direct government regulation enforced through the courts (Better regulation task force 2000a; National Consumer Council 1999). The key issue facing governments in regulating health care, as with other industries that employ professionals, is that professional practice requires a high level of expertise to regulate it appropriately. Government simply does not have enough expertise to regulate health care by itself.

> In complex areas where the Government does not have adequate expertise, any state solution may be significantly less effective than alternative approaches . . . The state should explore options for harnessing the existing expertise in an industry or profession. If the state chooses not to, it may encounter very effective blocks to enforcing its regulations as it may be starting from a lower knowledge base and find itself a step behind developments external to it.
> (Better regulation task force 2000a para 5.1.4)

A midway point between total government regulation and self-regulation is co-regulation, which refers to a situation where the regulatory role is shared between government and an industry body (Ministry of Commerce New Zealand 1999 para 54). Co-regulation can range from a simple endorsement of industry self-regulation to providing legislative backing to privately-defined rules when industry lacks sufficient sanctions to ensure compliance (thus bordering on traditional regulation) (Ayers and Braithwaite 1992). In general, co-regulation tends to mean the production of a set of general standards for the conduct of the trade or business (Better regulation task force 2003 page 45). An example of an area where co-regulation would be appropriate is in the area of General Medical Practice. 'The complex relationships between individual and collective interests in the services provided by Government through GPs suggest that this is an area where co-regulation should be developed which in turn means that interested groups should have an equal voice in regulatory bodies' (Better regulation task force 2000a para 4.4.2.2). The alternative is what has been termed enforced self-regulation, in which regulatory functions are subcontracted by the state to private commercial organizations. If the interested parties do not agree their own rules to the satisfaction of the state, the state can intervene with its own less tailored rules (Ayers and Braithwaite 1992).

A national, state-run regulatory body would not assist health care organizations to accept the challenge of innovation and modernization, nor to take on the additional challenge of self-governance required under devolved management. The fundamental problems of producing high quality health care cannot easily be addressed by central control.

> Quality has re-emerged as a sentinel issue in the field of health care delivery. Hospitals are being challenged by increasingly competitive market conditions and regulatory changes to produce high-quality care without raising health care costs. Moreover, hospital leaders face the additional challenge of developing policies, procedures and incentives to improve quality within a domain that has traditionally been the province of highly autonomous, professionally trained physicians. Responsibility for developing and overseeing these efforts rests first and foremost with the hospital governing board, the organisational entity held legally accountable for quality of care.
>
> (Weiner and Alexander 1993 page 375)

The UK government has proved reluctant to let go of responsibility for the NHS entirely, although it has recognized that some form of self-regulation is necessary to promote devolved management. Therefore, it was necessary for the government to introduce an independent body which would mimic a form of co-regulation but which would be funded by central government and would report to Parliament. The creation of Foundation Trusts went hand-in-hand with both the introduction of a new inspectorate, the Healthcare Commission, to inspect the quality of the systems of health care, and also the introduction of performance contracts setting out local standards and targets agreed with primary care trusts. However, it has been argued that the approach to central performance management, traditionally undertaken using large numbers of detailed performance targets, should change. The reasons given are twofold: first, it is held to be too dirigiste for devolved management; and second, it is considered to be an inappropriate form of control in a devolved system as complex and behaviourally dependent at health care.

The arguments against the use of central performance measures are based on the assumption that performance measures are a form of output control, stipulating what is required as the outcome of actions of organizations and their staff. Most performance measures are stated in terms of process outcomes, such as waiting lists and waiting times. This is driven in part by a belief that this is what the public wishes to assess, and in part by the great difficulty experienced in devising appropriate measures for clinical outcomes that contain high degrees of uncertainty. This questions the extent to which such output-based performance measures are capable of delivering the much sought after accountability. Evidence to-date suggests that, in general, members of the public do not understand indicators. Bruce Vladeck, a USA academic noted for his thinking on these topics, claimed the choice of performance measures is frequently akin to the drunk looking under the lamp-post for his car keys, not because the keys were dropped there but because it is the only place there is any light (Vladeck 1988). The general public, it could be argued, is under a different lamp-post from most people constructing performance management statistics. Furthermore, Berwick has pointed out that the production of performance measures does not necessarily result in improvements in care. 'The danger lies in a naïve and atheoretical belief rampant in the orgy of measurement involved in health care regulation, that the assessment and publication of performance data will somehow induce otherwise indolent care givers to improve the level of their care and efficiency' (Berwick 1989 page 55). This argument suggests that these outcome measures address the wrong sorts of controls.

Agency theory can lead to a questioning of the appropriateness of performance measures. If the model of the relationship between government and the Foundation Trusts is defined in terms of an agency relationship between the government, the principal and the hospital (the agent), there are indeed arguments in favour of outcome-based contracts. When the contract (social or implied) is between a principal and an agent and is outcome based, the agent is more likely to behave in the interest of the principal (Hood, James and Scott 2003). That is, the agent, in this case the Foundation Trust, will attempt to deliver what is required in performance terms. The natural consequence of a focus on performance is, however, exactly what devolution is intended to reverse – the organization becomes risk averse and avoids making changes which might prejudice the outcomes on which it is judged. If the purpose of devolution is to promote modernization through innovation, there is a need to transfer risk taking from the principal to the agent, to promote greater localized risk taking. The controls, therefore, should focus on behaviour rather than on outcomes. However, this requires considerable trust between the various parties involved. The situation becomes more complex when the governance arrangements are extended from simple accountability to central government to accountability to local constituencies, that is stakeholders.

Stakeholder models of governance are increasingly promoted as concerns about public mistrust of services have grown (O'Neill 2002; Power 1997). It is part of the logic behind the need for devolution of decision making to local communities, to replace the autocracy associated with central government with a reduction in state control. This has resulted in the rejection of old models of regulation, which are seen as remote and dictatorial.

> The UK's regulatory culture is inherently autocratic, inflexible and remote. This culture can be synonymous with totalitarianism, as in the old Soviet Union, or it can be benignly autocratic as during the crisis war years in Britain when, because of the external threat, citizens were happy to allow unprecedented state regulation in their

lives. But today's dilemma is that the lack of an external threat has transformed public attitudes from unquestioning trust and respect for government and professionals to cynicism and suspicion.

(Better regulation task force 2001 page 3)

Lord Irvine of Lairg, the Lord Chancellor, commented in a similar vein.

The world's democracies face many challenges in common. Public disillusionment with politics is one of the most critical. From country to country, our circumstances may differ, but we share a common challenge – the perception by people that government serves the governors, not the people . . . The United Kingdom has suffered from a long drift towards ever greater centralisation of political power. This has caused many to feel that they have little or no opportunity to influence the important decisions that affect their daily lives. The accountability of government to the people has been damaged by a culture of secrecy . . . Our solutions are based on the incremental development of a mature democracy, where government is brought closer to the people.

(Lord Irvine of Lairg 1999 quoted in Scott 2000)

In 1999, a MORI/BRU poll demonstrated that the public (as represented by ninety per cent of their sample of 1015 British adult respondents) wanted more openness in how the government makes its decisions. Indeed, a poll conducted in 2002 demonstrated that whereas ninety one per cent of those interviewed felt that they would trust doctors to tell the truth, only 20 per cent felt that they would trust government ministers to tell the truth (Cabinet Office 2002 page 35). 'The importance of trust in providing information is also crucial, both in terms of the believing the truthfulness of the source communicating the risk, but also in terms of having confidence that they can and will act to reduce the risk (which in turn will be linked to one's social and political beliefs)' (Cabinet Office 2002 annexes page 34).

Accountability, therefore, is related to the level of trust in society towards government and its institutions. Loss of trust, it is claimed, will prevent modernization. More importantly, it will cause the public and service users to disengage and not want to participate in service delivery. Building trust therefore requires the demonstration that decision making is open and also enables local participation in decision making and also the local scrutiny of the delivery of services.

Public sector bodies must combine reliable information produced by 'hard' systems and processes with the 'softer' issues of openness and integrity to inform their judgement on key decisions. The more open

and honest organisations are with themselves about their performance, the more open and honest they can be with service users and
the public.

(Audit Commission 2003 page 9)

The NHS already has organizational structures that incorporate corporate governance approaches through the existence of boards which run local health
services. However, the experience from private business has demonstrated that
the concentration of power in the hands of a few individuals in the organization's management or the board does not dispel concerns about trust and
accountability. This derives from the development of commercialism at the
beginning of the industrial revolution when firms were family owned and
there was a tendency towards what Wheeler and Silanpaa refer to as
unaccountable autocracy (Wheeler and Silanpaa 1997). They describe autocracy as being associated with paternalism and philanthropy – one individual
caring enough about his or her family of stakeholders to do the right thing by
all of them. And today it is associated with 'individual aggrandizement, tough
decisions and fabulous remuneration' (Wheeler and Silanpaa 1997 page 143).
In the public sector, it is also described as the frustration of a few people taking
decisions about people's lives and the use of public money, and this applies to
the structure of NHS boards as much as to other public services. However, the
loss of trust is not as simple as saying public services are failing (O'Neill 2002).
The relationship between the public and the services has changed. The public,
as both citizens and consumers, has greater access to education, knowledge
and information and has higher expectations of public services and can feel let
down when these are not provided.

The failure of public sector organizations to hold themselves appropriately to account has been thought to have created what has been called the
'blame culture'. The public, failing to have their demands for accountability
met by existing governance structures have begun to use the rapidly developing public media to broadcast management failure far and wide. 'In this
environment, the victims of bad management resort freely to the media in its
watchdog role. Arguably this has produced a form of accountability which is
acceptable to the public particularly because it is speedy and cheap and it puts
in place a means of redress which top management is beginning to respect'
(Mackay and Sweeting 2000 page 369). However, research conducted for the
health and safety executive and other departments suggests that although the
media can simplify and amplify risks, they can only amplify a risk if it reson-
ates with an existing public mood (Cabinet Office 2002; Petts, Horlick-Jones,
and Murdoch 2001). The public has, therefore, extended the concept of
accountability 'much further than the very ordered notion of legal accountability into the realm of public accountability which knows fewer bounds'
(Mackay and Sweeting 2000 page 269).

The role of stakeholders

The appeal of the stakeholder model to proponents of devolved governance is that it promotes participation and inclusiveness, thereby offering a broadened model of accountability based on greater opportunities for local people or their representatives to hold public services to account. Using arguments of democracy and citizen involvement, public sector stakeholding 'takes us into the territory of psychological contracts, trust, loyalty and inclusion'. Account-ability, in this context therefore, 'implies a social framework. Psychological and social norms precede organisational and institutional requirements. Accountability implies both a shared set of expectations and a common currency of justifications' (Day and Klein 1987 page 5).

In the stakeholding model, it is not enough to permit government to negotiate the shared set of expectations on behalf of local publics. Instead, there is the requirement to permit localized assessment and judgement of the performance of public services. New models of accountability, therefore, must recognize the requirements of devolution, requiring stronger self-determination by local communities, and must recognize the inherent com-plexity in the provision of health care involving many different organizations and multiple governance structures. Complexity can only be managed through complexity (Ashby 1968). Complex organizations and/or those oper-ating in a complex dynamic environment require complex control systems. This might be reflected in a compound board and/or a network of firms (Craven, Piercy and Shipp 1996) and/or by involving strategic stakeholders in the control of a firm (Blair 1995).

It is also necessary to ensure that information is produced that will enable the local stakeholders to judge the provision of health services. 'The cybernetic concept of feedback is a condition precedent for self-regulation or self-governance' (Ashby 1968 page 53). If a firm is not to affect adversely its stake-holders through its actions or inactions (Donaldson and Preston 1995), it will require governance processes that allow its stakeholders to participate in estab-lishing the appropriate methods for judging the quality of health services. In the case of health care, this would be the local public and its representatives (be they local authorities or local groups representing the local public) who need to be the main judges of the performance of the local organization (Wheeler and Silanpaa 1997). Hence the substantiation of the primary argu-ment behind the introduction of Foundation Trusts. In addition, a key feature of local governance is that local stakeholders need a power base independent of management, to protect them from being treated as whistle blowers. They must be accorded a local presence, a factor which is enshrined in the governance arrangements of these new organizations.

The model of accountability has to recognize that quality is a set of judgements made about various aspects of care. Based on Donabedian's categorization of quality into the elements of a system, inputs, processes and outputs, there are a number of different dimensions to quality that the public is interested in, when holding public sector managers to account. The first concentrates on examining the characteristics of the settings in which the care is provided (structure); the second examines the attributes of the process of care; and the third requires consideration of the overall impact of health care systems on the general population, such as in mortality and disease rates experienced in the population. Satisfaction with health care services is also seen as an important indicator of how well a health care system serves its population (Houses of the Oireachtais 2002). However, as discussed in Chapter 1, if the expectations of the public change and the culture of the health care organization does not change correspondingly, not only will satisfaction with the service reduce, so will its image in the eyes of the public and trust in the service will be undermined.

It is therefore necessary to find the appropriate combination of approaches to control which will meet the complex requirements of assessing health care for accountability purposes. There is a need to develop locally- based performance assessment regimes in which local health care organizations can be held to account through a national framework. An emphasis on innovation requires governance approaches that can allow intelligence and direction to emerge from continuing organization processes, in contrast with traditional approaches to planning which tend to impose goals, objectives and targets. This will require behavioural controls that can be negotiated locally and which can be used to ensure accountability for processes and a better understanding of how systems behave and need to be performance managed. 'Cybernetics also emphasizes the central role played by norms and standards (i.e. policies, procedures, indicators etc) as guidelines for action. It shows us that these guidelines are of significance as limits to be placed on system behaviour, rather than as specific targets to be achieved' (Wheeler and Silanpaa 1997 page 131).

Standardization

The earlier aims of the NHS were to produce a uniformly available health service of uniform quality. This has been dismissed by some as a myth. The pursuit of uniformity, it is claimed, has had 'a uniquely detrimental impact on standards, in discouraging initiative, innovation and improvement. To this extent diversity is strength. A great diversity of ways to deliver healthcare is what is needed' (Lea and Mayo 2002 page 14). Diversity, recognizing local differences, is held to be central to encouraging innovation. The new approach to governance has, therefore, to be able to permit local flexibility in service provision, local accountability in negotiating judgements of process and outcome and yet at the same time, to ensure equity and standardization of quality. That is, there is a need for the simultaneous achievement of local flexibility in delivery and yet uniformity in quality.

One solution to this has been that there should be national standards within a regulatory framework which 'clarifies for patients what they can expect and gives them effective management, leadership and accountability' (Department of Health 2002b Para 1.13).

> There must be a single, coherent, co-ordinated set of generic standards: that is, standards relating to the patient's experience and the systems for ensuring that care is safe and of good quality (for example corporate management, clinical governance, risk management, clinical audit, the management and support of staff, and the management of resources). Trusts must comply with these standards.
>
> (Department of Health 2002b page 59)

It is significant who sets the standards in a system of health care in which management is devolved and which depends upon inspection to provide assurance that quality services are provided. The use of national standards to develop a framework to assess the quality of health care has occurred in a number of countries. In France, the government has adopted a national accreditation programme. In Scotland, the clinical standards board assesses health care organizations against agreed upon standards. In both cases, the inspectorates act as agents of the government. However, this potentially can create difficulties for governments, particularly as in the case of the NHS, when the government is held responsible for the direct provision of health care. When inspectorates are created as an instrument of government, but also given independence, the inspectorate potentially has the power to define the quality of health care: 'Criteria and standards are also powerful instruments of professional and political control: those who control the criteria and standards have the whole of health care in their thrall' (Donabedian 1988a page 181). In a devolved management system, standards have to be flexible enough to allow the local determination of objectives – thereby allowing for local differences in the design and structure of delivery systems – but at the same time have a standard approach to quality, particularly of clinical care. This is important when equity and fairness in the receipt of health care is part of the assumptions about the nature of quality of health care. 'In the past there were no national standards; there was almost complete professional autonomy for clinicians; and different levels of care were provided in different parts of the country. As a result there were confused accountabilities and a lottery of care for the individual patient' (Department of Health 2002b para 1.13).

Traditional forms of external review lead inevitably to the development of detailed organizational criteria to aid the process of inspection. Detailed criteria permit non-experts to undertake assessments. They stop criticisms of bias in the judgement of inspectors because they specify precisely what is required. Staff follow the instructions provided and this leads to standardization of processes and procedures. However, detailed criteria present difficulties in a health care system which is striving to reform its structure and its practices. They frequently create what can be described as an organizational straight-jacket, which restricts organizations from following the requirements spelt out in the criteria. From the logic of devolved management, to create the health care systems required by today's public and politicians, it follows that intelligent and creative management is required, which in turn calls for a new approach to inspection. This would require that inspectors are skilled in a more judgemental approach, which would be capable of withstanding the criticism of bias. In this approach, inspectors would have to use 'intelligent assessment' based on what Sir Ian Kennedy has described as 'intelligent information'. But in order to limit the function of the inspectorate to providing assurance to the public, patients and service users, the government would have to determine not only the framework of the universally accepted definition of quality, that is the standards, but also to decide the appropriateness and the acceptability of the forms of audit and inspection used, that is the criteria used and the method of assessment employed against them.

National standards to encourage local development would have to be capable of being applied across the country, be acceptable to professionals and patients, and create the control systems which reflect the values chosen to underpin the health system.

> National standards of clinical care should reflect the commitment to patient-centred care and thus in future be formulated from the perspective of the patient. The standards should address the quality of care that a patient with a given illness or condition is entitled to expect to receive from the NHS. The standards should take account of the best available evidence. The standards should include guidance on how promptly patients should get access to care. They should address the roles and responsibilities of the various healthcare professionals who will care for the patient. They should take account of the patient's journey from primary care, into the hospital system (if necessary), and back to primary and community care, and of the necessary facilities and equipment.
>
> (The Report of the Public Inquiry into children's heart surgery at the Bristol Royal Infirmary 1984–1995 2001 page 126)

Independent inspection would reveal lack of compliance with the standards and would enable the construction of action plans to achieve compliance with the standards. Any regulatory action taken towards organizations that did not comply would have to contain sanctions to encourage compliance, as well as incentives to reward and encourage progress.

The standards that were produced, referred to as the 'Standards for Better Health', resembled many other organizational standards found around the world, reflecting what are universally accepted definitions of good structural elements for health care (Department of Health 2004). However, they were unusual in that they described the elements of a health care system rather than specifying the processes required for health care. They focused on the key components of safe, clinically effective, patient-centred health care; good governance; and accessible and responsive care. Although not new in their prominence as elements of modern health care, they were the distillation of good practice recognized internationally, which had been enshrined in earlier Department of Health policy documents.

To be truly modern, health care systems need to become more flexible, to allow services to meet rapidly changing needs and new developments in clinical care. Standards suitable for encouraging flexibility cannot dictate the structure of, for example, a good infection control system, for this needs to vary according to the circumstances of individual patients and the work of individual organizations, including the nature and the structure of the buildings in which services are provided. The 'Standards for Better Health' recognized that there cannot be an assumption of a single prescription of good practice, but that there are universally-recognized values and assumptions about good quality in health care, which need to be continuously restated and reinforced through external review. The standards were written intentionally to be high level, reflecting policy and not management requirements which, in theory, allowed for assessment criteria to be tailored to recognize local conditions and differences between services and population, patient and user groups.

Standards can be used in two ways. The first is to produce a consensus on the features of good quality in health care. The second is to create a framework for an inspection process in which external reviewers determine whether the standards are complied with. In turn, the findings from inspection can be used to generate a mechanism for licencing; that is, failure to comply with the standards will cause a health care facility to be closed down or refused entry into the market. In addition the standards set the minimum requirements placed on an organization to ensure it is able to function safely. Brennan and Berwick define this mechanism as the culling of organisations (Brennan and Berwick 1995). Alternatively, inspection findings can be used for certification, in that the supply of, for example, NHS funds could be denied to an organization that failed to meet the standard-defining quality. Or standards can be used to demonstrate good practice, set at a higher level than most organizations can achieve, providing a level to which they can aspire.

There are different arguments as to which of these models is most appropriate for health care. Berwick has argued that although professionals

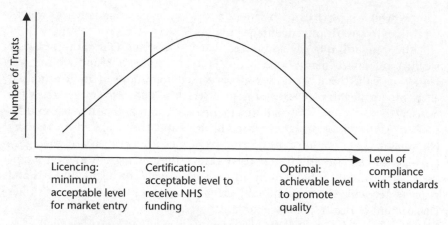

Figure 6.1 Use of assessments of compliance with standards.

must take part in specifying preferred methods of care, they should avoid the search for minimalist standards of care, which normally accompanies inspection to improve quality. The specification of minimum standards for structure, process or outcome rapidly change from being 'floors to ceilings' and become seen as the acceptable level of achievement. However, 'specifications of process (clear, scientifically grounded, continuously reviewed statements of how one intends to behave) are essential to quality improvement and are widely lacking in health care' (Berwick 1989 page 56).

The choice of organizationally-based standards as opposed to clinically-driven concerns is a familiar one in the design of standards-based assessment systems. There are different schools of thought as to the purpose of standards and what they can be expected to achieve. Standards are mainly used to describe and to assess what a health care organization is 'capable of', that is what it is designed to achieve, rather than what it actually does achieve. The emphasis, therefore, is on appropriate organizational design rather than on the achievement of specific clinical outcomes or behaviours on the part of staff. Assessment against a standard can most easily assess whether policies and procedures are in place, rather than whether they are used. This is the argument behind the adherence to the principles of Continuous Quality Improvement in standards setting. The purpose of quality-improvement-based standards is to assess whether the organization is well designed and capable of achievement, rather than the guarantee that it will achieve good quality. So a standard can be written, for example, to ensure that performance statistics are reviewed regularly. What it cannot guarantee is that regular review will result in better clinical care. However, it can provide assurance that the management and clinicians were doing their best to comply with the review requirements.

Most standards-based systems are designed to describe the environment in which clinical care can flourish, rather than addressing specific requirements of clinical care. There is little evidence to demonstrate that organizational standards do directly result in improved clinical care. Rather, they provide an environment that does not hamper the delivery of good clinical care. However, recent research evidence from the USA has demonstrated that accreditation (by the Joint Commission on Accreditation of Healthcare Organisations (JCAHO)) does provide some information concerning hospitals' quality of care and outcomes in the aggregate. Indeed, knowing that a hospital participated in the JCAHO process suggests superior quality and outcomes compared with non-surveyed hospitals. It is unknown, however, whether the process of undergoing JCAHO accreditation improves the quality of care or whether this association reflects self-selection against JCAHO evaluation by more poorly performing hospitals. However,

> many of the JCAHO standards do not assess quality in day-to-day patient care activities. For example, a high degree of compliance with administrative or managerial standards is unlikely to have much bearing on whether patients receive aspirin on admission for AMI. Identifying hospitals that are well managed, while informative, is likely to be different than identifying hospitals that provide high-quality clinical care.
>
> (Chen et al. 2003 page 250)

Where generic standards have been developed to work alongside organizational or disease or condition specific standards, the standards tend now to reflect factors affecting the experience of patients. This is the case in the NHS with the development of the standards included in the National Service Frameworks, which describe the key issues in the care of specific groups of patients, such as the elderly, children or those suffering from cancer, heart disease or diabetes. Frequently the design of standards will be based upon selected principles, which can be used to provide a structure around which the standards can be organized. For example, New Zealand Quality Health emphasizes that providers need to understand the needs and preferences of the client and family, and the client needs to understand the options and shares in decision making. In their definition, responsiveness includes the concepts of acceptability and participation. This leads them to conclude that a responsive service is one that provides respect for persons and is client orientated. This is based upon the assumptions that: respect for persons includes respect for their dignity, confidentiality and autonomy to participate in choices about their health and support; and client orientation includes prompt attention, facilities and amenities of adequate quality, access to social support networks and choice of service provider.

The original model for organizational standards, established by the Joint Commission on Accreditation of Healthcare Organisations (JCAHO) in the United States, contained standards that were devised to describe the organization of hospital services – the main features of hospital departments. From five standards developed in 1918, the number of standards to describe a hospital rose to over 4000 by the early 1990s. At this time, it was realized that there were too many standards in use and effort was directed at reducing the number of standards. In addition, as the emphasis on hospital care began to wane world wide and governments have been searching for other ways to provide health care, there has been a rapid growth in the other areas to which standards could be directed, such as mental health services, ambulatory care, trauma services, etc. There have been three other developments that have impacted upon the development of standards. First, the development of commissioning – the purchaser-provider split has resulted in standards for commissioning organizations commonly referred to as network standards as they cover the relationships between funding and providing organizations. Second, there is a world-wide retreat from the direct provision of services by governments, which has led to greater interest in the development of standards that monitor the outcomes of health care. Third, there has been a desire to create standards that reflect more than just the organizational and structural aspects of health care, resulting in the development of disease group focused standards, such as those for diabetes, etc. Many standards-based systems have been attempting to integrate the management of clinical processes into the organizational standards.

However, the standards for better health developed for the National Health Service were designed to perform a different function. They were to lay the foundations for the development of assessment processes and, therefore, could not be restricted to specific clinical considerations. The NHS already had sets of standards in the National Service Frameworks, which described the requirements for groups of patients. The new standards were to be generic standards describing the workings of the whole health care system. Furthermore, they were not intended to be the basis for organizational audit. They did not prescribe how organizations should be organized and run, by providing checklists which could be ticked off by auditors.

Sir Ian Kennedy, in his report on the factors surrounding the deaths of children at the Bristol Royal Infirmary, argued that there should be two types of standards – those that address issues which are obligatory and must be observed and those to which the NHS should aspire over time (The Report of the Public Inquiry into children's heart surgery at the Bristol Royal Infirmary 1984–1995 2001). This reveals an interesting issue in the debate about the control of quality through standards. To what extent must standards reflect a static view of health care, or can quality improvement be written into the standards or achieved through either ratcheting up the standards or the assessment criteria over time? Modern thinking about health care suggests that there is a need for quality to reflect integrated working between health care organizations and an implicit focus on the patient experience of health services. These require standards that address implicitly and explicitly issues of patient choice, service redesign, and making the best use of scarce skills. It is not clear whether modern ideas about quality in health care can be successfully enshrined in static indicators of quality which describe the 'features of the physical and organisational structure of the institution' (Donabedian 1986 page 107). Is it possible to select a baseline of mandatory features with which health care institutions must comply, which do not define health care organizations in such a way as to prevent the organizations themselves from changing their design and function to meet changing patient and societal needs? To permit flexibility in the design of services and continuous enhancement of service provision, standards must be written in such a way as to provide incentives for organizations to seek out opportunities for improvement in the design and functioning of services within the whole health care system (Department of Health 2004). To capture the new thinking about health care, standards need to recognize the synergy between the different elements of health care that contribute to quality. Therefore, national standards should provide a single focus for the quality of health care for the whole complex system of health care, made up of many organizations, professionals and patients.

Inspection and audit

Inspection is a process of periodic, targeted scrutiny, used to provide an independent check and to report on whether services are meeting national and local performance standards, legislative and professional requirements and the needs of service users (Public Audit Forum 2001). The primary role of inspectors is to promote accountability – by informing the public and government about the current quality of services and their potential for improvement. With the focus on quality, they can be an instrument of change 'by holding up an external and objective mirror to the inspected body, helping it to identify priorities for improvement, and challenging poor performance' (Public Audit Forum 2002 Para 12). Inspectors frequently make recommendations in their reports, thus promoting good practice. However, in this circumstance the inspection body defines the practices and procedures within an organization, using centrally-agreed models of good practice and frequently this conflicts with the notion of independent and devolved management.

Inspection can be conducted in a number of different ways but in the main there are two types of inspection: that conducted by full-time paid inspectors and peer review. Peer review uses professionals employed within service delivery organizations and is often recommended as a means to ensure continuous learning and improvement using standards (Strategic policy making team, Cabinet office 1999 para 1.4). The main aim of this form of inspection is to ensure that national standards are consistently applied across organizations. For example, in the case of health care it is argued that patients have a right to adequate services from all health care professionals. 'To ensure that there are consistent standards, GPs must monitor each other in partnership practices and steps must be taken to ensure that single doctor practices meet the same standards' (Better regulation task force 2000a para 4.4.2.5). Peer review is, therefore, a form of monitoring against standards which is less threatening than official inspection, because it is conducted by peers who should be sympathetic, although independent, and can provide support to the professionals they are reviewing.

Inspection can, therefore, provide assurance in that it checks whether services are meeting the needs of service users and are achieving levels of performance consistent with national and local performance standards and targets. In doing this, it can also provide assurance on the 'economy, efficiency and effectiveness with which resources are used in meeting professional and service standards' (Public Audit Forum 2001 para 30). The difficulty encountered is that not only can the inspection process reduce management autonomy, it is also the case that inspectors are known to be variable in their assessments, frequently using discretion in their visits as to the areas and the potential problems they examine. The Joint Commission on Accreditation of Healthcare Organisations has admitted that assessment can be subjective and 'the impact of the variation by and between observers is unknown' (Chen *et al.* 2003 page 251). This was demonstrated by the awards given for assessed compliance with their standards. 'The distinction between those who get commendation and those who fall just short is artificial' (Moore 1999 page 15).

While inspection has traditionally focused on organizational systems and processes, rather than the assessment of internal control systems, audit has usually been the mechanism for examining internal controls (Vass and Simmonds 2001a page 13). However, audit is more associated with stewardship of resources, whereas inspection traditionally is primarily concerned with 'professional and service standards' (Public Audit Forum 2002 para 65). The audit approach to internal control has, therefore, not evolved to monitor service quality and so struggles to deliver an assessment of organization-wide control systems in organizations as complex as hospitals or primary care. Auditors tend to focus on specific aspects of an organization. Financial audit, for example, provides assurance on the accounts and the financial aspects of corporate governance, and on those aspects of corporate governance that relate to performance management, and on the use of resources including performance information systems (Public Audit Forum 2002 para 29).

Auditors' role is to identify and report weaknesses in, amongst other things, financially-related internal controls (Public Audit Forum 2002). There is a branch of audit that focuses primarily on internal control systems, to evaluate how adequate and effective they are. The primary focus of this audit is not public accountability but to assist management in the effective discharge of their duties and responsibilities. Internal auditors are employees of the organization and their task is to help their organization accomplish its objectives by bringing a systematic, disciplined approach to the evaluation and improvement of risk management activities, control activities and governance processes. Internal auditing reviews the reliability and integrity of information, compliance with policies and regulations, the safeguarding of assets, the economical and efficient use of resources, and established operational goals and objectives. Internal control systems are continuously changing as the work undertaken and the technology used within organizations changes. The task of internal auditors is to monitor the control systems and to judge their adequacy for managing the risks the organization faces.

Auditors tend to use what are referred to as substantive tests, which are tests of details and analytical procedures performed to detect material misstatements in financial reporting. These would include examination of such things as: a manager's review of purchases prior to approval (preventing inappropriate expenditures of office funds) or whether a computer program that asks for a password prevents unauthorized access to information.

> Performance auditors and inspectors judge the performance of the service, government programme, function or transaction under review against best practice (or where no external comparator is available, normative criteria) established by national research and evidence collected from previous audits and inspections.
>
> (Public Audit Forum 2002 para 34)

Again, this contrasts with the work of inspectors who tend to use checklists and standards to identify organizational features or systems. However, management auditors have tended to drift into using inspection-style checklists to help them assess organizations, with the inevitable result that when audit has attempted in the past to address issues of service quality, it has begun to look like inspection. The boundaries between audit and inspection have become blurred and frequently organizations subjected to audit and inspection regimes cannot see a difference in the approaches – they both seem as onerous as each other and remarkably similar in their conduct. Indeed, so similar have the functions become that the word audit is frequently used as an equivalent to monitoring, and can 'encompass many forms of review, inspection and certification, whether formal or informal, or involving internal or external reporting' (Vass and Simmonds 2001a page 2).

Inspection and audit, although they have different origins, appear over time to have converged as regulatory instruments. The main characteristic of their activity in the public sector 'is their independence in judgement' (Public Audit Forum 2002 para 24), which is the main reason for both claiming to be able to support the delivery of accountability. But neither have evolved well enough to develop into a system that can offer adequate accountability within a devolved infrastructure. Both have tended towards becoming central regulators. Different bodies, whether referred to as inspectors or auditors, for a variety of reasons have been given different powers to act as regulators, that is to impose controls and behaviour change on organizations.

> While auditors and inspectors rely mainly on the publications of findings to drive change and improve performance, regulators have executive powers to secure compliance. Some inspectors also have the power to recommend the transfer of functions or even prevent bodies from operating where standards are deemed to be unacceptably low. However where inspectors exercise these powers they could be seen as acting as a regulator of the body under review.
>
> (Public Audit Forum 2002)

Even though audit and inspection have tried to develop in order to deal with issues of service quality, they are felt in general to be too heavy-handed and inappropriate to promote the twin objectives of modern health care: the devolution of power away from central control; and the encouragement of well managed risk taking to ensure continuous innovation and improvement. Furthermore, the costs and the burdens of traditional audit and inspection are felt to be too great and government is seeking to move away from the culture of over-inspection in the public sector (Lord Sharman 2002; House of Commons 1999). In the past, this had led to the argument that there should be enforced self-regulation with more stringent audit or inspection for poorly-performing organizations. Ayres and Braithwaite (1992) suggest that a regulatory hierarchy can be created, which is designed to provide maximum incentives for early compliance. Organizations that 'resist early compliance will be pushed up the enforcement pyramid. Not only escalating penalties but also escalating frequency of inspection . . . can then negate the returns to delayed compliance' (Ayers and Braithwaite 1992 page 39). This message was translated into UK government policy for dealing with public sector organizations, and referred to as lighter touch regulation, which was defined as:

> Intervening in inverse proportion to success and striking an appropriate balance between intervening where services are failing and giving successful organisations the freedom to manage. In other words, the enforced self-regulation doctrine involves the deployment of heavier

regulatory tackle against the incompetent or recalcitrant while lightening the regulatory yoke over good performers.

(Vass and Simmonds 2001a page 12)

However, lighter touch regulation can only work when there is an acceptable system for determining which organisations are doing well and which are not. And as has already been established, this cannot be determined solely by performance or outcome measurements. Stakeholders and the local public need to be involved in determining the parameters of good quality and they also need to be involved in judging the quality of risk management with the organization. There is a need to find a method that assesses how well organizations are managed, to provide necessary public accountability and to justify intervention by regulators.

But in the search for a new approach to inspection, it has to be remembered that the state cannot act as an independent assessor to provide the objective assessment required for assurance. It is an interested party in regulation and, therefore, cannot be independent. And it does not have the expertise to deal with the complex issues of professional practice in the health service. Therefore, independent review has to be conducted by a third party.

Central government, in its search for standardization of the provision of services, has tended to support the use of audit and inspection as the tools which generate compliance with centrally-determined requirements. In this respect, governments are seeking solace in a battery of regulatory armaments to enforce a central view of good behaviour. As Braithwaite points out 'much of the academic debate about enforcement revolves around the distinction between deterrence and compliance' (Brennan and Berwick 1995 page 21). The deterrence model is founded on the belief that the regulated concerns must be given firm rules, not advice. Advocates of compliance, on the other hand, take a gentler view that regulation should be largely a matter of persuasion. The former belief leads to tough inspectors with strong sanctioning authority. The latter approach leads to a major role for regulators as consultants. But of course, persuasive regulators can be co-opted by the very organizations they seek to regulate, a condition known as regulatory capture. If inspection is undertaken by an independent self-regulatory body, it will, inevitably, be part of the community which is interpreting the changes that are taking place in the external environment. The greater the shared understanding between the inspectorate and the inspected, in terms of norms, standards and definitions, the less rules have to be made explicit and there is less need for precision in the writing of rules to control behaviour (Black 1997 page 35). This reduces the need for documentation, but increases the likelihood of charges of collusion between the inspectors and the inspected. It is difficult to work with organizations to try to improve quality while maintaining the necessary independence to achieve public accountability (Brennan and Berwick 1995 page 21).

The example frequently cited is that of the Joint Commission on Accreditation of Healthcare Organisations (JCAHO):

> The JCAHO history captures the spirit of regulation in health care. First it was dominated by an ascendant profession and in many ways reinforced the primacy of the physician's role in determining quality. Second, and as a result, JCAHO rules did not evince an external rationality. Instead the organisation fell into a rather meaningless mode of external inspection that suited most parties . . . Indeed one could predict that if the JCAHO were to demonstrate independence, the hospital industry and medical profession would probably interpret this as antagonism.
>
> (Brennan and Berwick 1995 page 44)

There are two other behavioural effects that have been observed when inspections take place, referred to as colonization and decoupling (Power 1997). Colonization occurs when inspectors' values and interests begin to supplant those of the inspected. This causes the bureaucratization of the inspection process. 'Organisations start to focus upon documenting processes and levels of direct output rather than results in outcome terms. This may be particularly the case where review tends to be compliance focused' (Vass and Simmonds 2001b page 3). Associated with this can be the production of data solely for the purpose of the review. The focus on approved processes demanded by the inspectors can displace more effective efforts to achieve quality improvement. Decoupling occurs when the impact of reviews is deliberately marginalized. The review activity is treated more as a ceremony or a ritual than as having any direct impact on the working of the organization (Power 1997).

Most external review processes are incapable of restricting themselves to simply monitoring health care organizations. Most attempt to create changes in the health care organizations, through forcing them to follow the model of good practice on which the design of the organizational standards that underpin the assessment process was based. This is because without the justification of promoting good practice and improvement, few bodies that monitor quality can justify their existence. 'Monitoring to have a purpose must be associated with mechanisms for control and enforcement whether direct or indirect' (Vass and Simmonds 2001a page 4). The model of change that most external review systems espouse is that of continuous quality improvement. Continuous quality improvement is a method of approaching management improvement. It is normally associated with the development of internal management processes. However, there has been a desire in recent times for governments to believe that they can drive continuous improvement from the centre, which has led to particular problems with the conduct of regulation.

The role of external review bodies and inspectorates has extended in recent years however with the development of continuous improvement and their use of incentives particularly publicity and league tables. These incentives become a mechanism for indirect enforcement and therefore the line between external review bodies and regulators becomes increasingly blurred.

(Vass and Simmonds 2001a page 4)

It is, therefore, generally assumed that external review bodies should either operate as regulators with enforcement power, or report to bodies who have policy and enforcement responsibilities. However, in a system of devolved management, where the power to control the health care system is truly given to organizations, it is necessary to divorce external review from regulation.

There is probably a case for separating out the culture of inspection, intended to provide independent quality assurance, from that of regulation. If the regulatory function of the Department were passed to a more formal regulator, accountable to the Secretary of State and to Parliament, the result would be a slimmer Department of Health, better integrated with devolved administrations, focused on policy development and acting as a strategic facilitator of the overall health system.

(Lea and Mayo 2002 page 25)

External review should, therefore, provide information to the bodies who are given the power to determine the acceptability of the quality of health care. This condition places a requirement on the system of external review to produce information about the organization rather than to encourage it to change from within itself.

Quality and regulation

Brennan and Berwick, in their review of the quality of regulation in health care in the United States, suggest two premises for future regulation. They argue that regulation should be assessed by the extent to which it accomplishes its social aims without compromising other important aims and without creating waste. Regulation, therefore, should be judged according to its outcomes. And second, that regulation should be responsive and collaborative for the good of patients. Responsive regulation is intended to reflect the structure of the industry being regulated, and to achieve its impact through encouraging self-regulation at the level of the processes and practices operated by the organizations and the people working within the system. Brennan and Berwick argue that inspection is a necessary part of responsive regulation but that current inspection approaches are 'among the worst known in any industry' (Brennan and Berwick 1995 page 364). Responsive regulation can, of itself, undermine the principles of devolution. The external review body becomes the judge and jury for the quality of health care provided rather than the devolved body to whom the power has been given. It is better to abandon inspection as regulation and to replace it with a system that is designed to follow more closely the principles of audit in providing assurance and accountability, rather than attempting to deliver improvement in the quality of health care as part of the inspection process.

Many of the features Brennan and Berwick (1995) identify as good practice in regulation are, in fact, good practice for external review in general, including the notion of not attempting to enforce behaviour change. They argue that regulators can only work with the ways in which the regulated can respond, that is, the ways in which providers can improve quality. They identify five different methods for improving quality. First, repairing, that is the ability of systems to repair and redress defects when they occur. Second, is culling or sorting, that is the assessment of performance and results with the purpose of removing services that fall below acceptable standards. Third, copying, by which organizations can learn to improve by copying others who are better. Improvement comes from standardizing processes or behaviours to conform to an ideal model. Fourth, learning in cycles, which is learning from changes made through innovation and experimentation in parts of the organization and spreading these practices to other parts of the organisation. Fifth and finally, creating, which is major change resulting from the development of a new technology, for example (Brennan and Berwick 1995).

Brennan and Berwick argue that inspection should accredit modern management and quality assurance processes and structures rather than examining the 'down-stream' results, that is, it should not be based on output controls. Continuous quality improvement can be addressed by examining the organization's approach to introducing continuous quality. Vass and Simmonds suggest that a distinction should be made between continuous improvement of standards themselves, and improvements in the cost-effective delivery of a set standard (Vass and Simmonds 2001a page 10). They also claim that health care regulation fails to identify explicit aims or goals for the health services it is regulating. 'We believe regulation would be better designed if all involved had a common set of measurable objectives' (Brennan and Berwick 1995 page 371). This is exacerbated when regulation attempts to address continuous quality improvement as it is too open-ended a goal to achieve accountability.

The role of fostering continuous improvement as noted above can be incorporated within the general framework but there needs to be clarity of objectives where review bodies play multiple roles and in particular where those roles have developed to include surrogate indirect enforcement mechanisms through incentives such as 'name and shame'.

(Vass and Simmonds 2001a page 10)

However, if the emphasis on regulation is removed from the Brennan and Berwick argument, what is left is a system that focuses on management and quality assurance processes and which addresses a common set of measurable objectives. If these arguments are taken in conjunction with the growing body of evidence that inspection as a form of health care regulation to improve quality is increasingly criticized as an ineffective method to improve quality (Donabedian 1980) and that most approaches to inspection of health care quality create an increasingly bureaucratic burden upon health care workers, especially clinicians (Jun, Peterson and Zsidisin 1998), then there is a strong case for a method of assessment that seeks to provide assurance based upon the examination of internal control systems.

Brennan and Berwick also argue for the need to focus on integrated systems and for the reduction in the extent of competition and duplication among regulators. Both of these are recognizable arguments in favour of examining control systems in devolved management systems. Integrated systems require partnerships and recognition of the difficulties in creating partnership controls that have to be negotiated between the various partners. Any consideration of regulatory processes in health care has to recognize the primacy of systems in the provision of health care.

Behavioural controls on information sharing, which creates mutual trust, are frequently the most appropriate controls for these forms of collaborative endeavour. Typical approaches to inspection of health care quality based upon standards that describe good organization cannot address the issues of behavioural controls. And the need for negotiated assessment, which must underpin the definition of acceptable behavioural controls, supports the case for a stakeholder approach to the agreeing and setting of controls. The only logical conclusion is that there has to be another approach to assessing the way in which health care organizations can be held to account for the quality of care for which they are responsible.

Chapter summary

This chapter has dealt with the following points:

- The issues surrounding devolved management.
- A description of different types of regulation.
- A discussion of the stakeholder model.
- The use of standards to achieve a uniform level of quality in health care.
- The processes of inspection and audit in the assessment of health care organizations.
- How to regulate for the highest possible level of quality.

7 New Governance and Intelligent Accountability

What form of governance is appropriate for a health care system in which management is devolved, with minimal central control in a world where the demands for accountability are high and the level of trust the public has for public services is low (O'Neill 2002; Strategy Unit 2002)? The arguments for reducing bureaucracy and reducing regulation are well rehearsed. In spite of this, there is considerable nervousness about deregulation. The experience from California, which went into a form of deregulation in its energy industry that substituted 'public monopolies' for 'private monopolies' (Clark and Bradshaw 2003), was felt directly to have contributed to the behaviour of the Enron corporation.

> Fully four years before (1997) the energy market in California was to be deregulated ... the California Public Utilities Commission ruled to move ahead in a unanimous decision to 'throw open the state's $20 billion electricity market to competition' to 'make California the first state to join a worldwide movement to deregulate utilities'.
>
> (Clark and Demirag 2002 p106)

The argument behind deregulation was the promotion of more competition between producers, lower prices, increasing consumer choice and increasing the reliability of services. The result was a crisis in the Californian energy industry. This led to a recommendation that there should be greater regulation, particularly for public services that supply key infrastructure for society (The Amazing Disintegrating Firm 2001). Clark and Demirag claim that one view of the cause of the Enron crisis came not from regulation or deregulation but from the economic theories that proposed reductions in government regulation, such as those promulgated by Michael Porter (1990), which failed to appreciate the significance of the maintenance of infrastructure to the running of society. This form of 'social contract' between a population and the market is held to be the role of government (Clark and Demirag 2002) and the case of

Enron proved that government involvement, rather than reducing the willingness of private organizations to take risks, is instead vital to those industries that provide critical social infrastructure. However, as has been pointed out, there is no evidence supporting the claims that deregulation was at fault. Deregulation had produced many advantages. Instead, a popularly held view has been that the spectacular failure of Enron was not the fault of the management, but the fault of those who were entrusted with delivering public accountability – the auditors. And therefore, it is the auditors who should be better regulated, rather than the industry.

> The first [priority] is the regulation of auditors. For years the profession has insisted that self-regulation and peer review are the right way to maintain standards. Yet Enron has shown that this is no longer enough . . . [The second priority] is the urgent need to eliminate conflicts of interest in accounting firms. Andersen collected audit fees of $25m from Enron, its second-biggest client, last year, but it earned even more for consulting and other work . . . [The final priority is] . . . America's accounting standards. GAAP [generally accepted accounting principles] standards used to be thought the most rigorous in the world. Yet under British standards [*sic*] Enron would not have been able to overstate its profits by so much.
>
> (Economist 2002)

Accountability and devolved power

Devolved power requires a strong accountability framework, capable of delivering the appropriate information to the public on the functioning of an organization. There is a vast array of methods in use to generate information for accountability purposes. A popular approach is the indirect assessment of care, which uses standards laid down for the appropriate structures of a health care organization. This is frequently conducted through what is termed accreditation, in which teams of reviewers or surveyors examine an organization for its level of compliance with published standards or inspection processes using the skilled judgement of independent reviewers. Alternatively, inspectors may be used to assess the internal mechanisms for ensuring that the care of patients conforms to expected, agreed upon processes, such as care pathways or other treatment schedules. In addition, central government monitoring of measures, such as the overall impact of health care systems on society, can be used – these examine the effects of care on the health and welfare of individuals or populations using measures such as mortality and disease rates. All are intended to provide reassurance to the public that health care services are well managed on their behalf.

Accountability demanded on this scale does not come free. The requirement to provide information incurs costs for those providing the information (Lord Sharman 2002 para 5.18). There have been attempts to co-ordinate programmes of inspection and audit to make them more coherent, thereby assisting with the production of information for accountability purposes (Lord Sharman 2002 para 5.23), and to reduce costs by relying on the work of other auditors and inspectors (HM Treasury 2002a para 2.45).

> It would be neither cost effective not fair and reasonable for all the bodies in the spending chain . . . to be constantly subject to several layers of audit. Efficiency requires that public auditors seek to maximize . . . the use they make of the work of others such as internal auditors, regulators and external auditors of related bodies.
>
> (Public Audit Forum 2000 para 20)

The single audit assumption, upon which much recent work of internal control has been predicated, emphasizes the need for a unified approach to the audit of public bodies, but more importantly, if emphasizes the need for a standardized approach to the provision of assurance through the standardization of assessment processes for examining the effectiveness of internal control.

Self-regulation

Health care professionals like to argue for self-regulatory models which allow their own kind to assess their own performance. Peer review enables a supportive emphasis on quality improvement, which reduces the threatening burdens imposed by regulatory audit. However, peer review is normally conducted to assess compliance with input-oriented standards (Scrivens 1995). The leadership of the Joint Commission on Accreditation of Healthcare Organisations realized that most of the measures of quality were primarily 'input-oriented' or focused on the structure of the institution – not just staff credentialing but all aspects of the institution. This was so because of the belief that 'there is a very high correlation between, on the one hand, a safe and functionally efficient physical plant, effectively qualified personnel, and properly developed procedures and, on the other hand, the quality of care provided to patients' (Jacobs, Chritoffel, and Dixon 1976). However, input-oriented standards, because they tend to be highly prescriptive, do not provide the kind of freedom and flexibility required to enable health care organizations to make changes and innovate.

Trust in professionals working in organizations requires that individuals act in predictable ways. And this has led to an assumption in the past that bureaucratic controls, which aim to standardize actions and behaviour are the best method of ensuring predictability. However, the increase in complexity of professional tasks, and the need for individuals to work in teams across organizational boundaries to deliver care means that trust cannot be delivered in traditional ways. The continuous change and redesign required by the modernization agenda, and the emphasis on life-long learning and re-skilling of professionals, means that health services are moving towards 'portfolio workers' (Handy 1994), thus requiring more flexible and individually-oriented forms of controls.

Furthermore, traditional accountability mechanisms, such as management structures and internal management reporting systems, not only fail to provide adequate information to the public about the quality of health care, but also have been found to discourage innovation and change because they tend to encourage risk aversion and lack incentives to manage risks. External review systems are frequently designed to reflect traditional approaches, with standards that reflect management and organizational structures. This is due in part to assumptions about the nature of accountability, but also derives from the fact that there is a shortage of competent auditors who can exercise independent judgement. External review systems are forced to structure their approach to assessment around prescriptive standards and checklists to assess compliance. This is the case even when external review is conducted as self-regulation, for example, by using accreditation systems (Scrivens 1995). Such standards are rarely designed to recognize the variety of approaches to service development that devolved power permits and they do not allow the recipients of services the opportunity to decide on the nature of the provision which they may enjoy. Nationally-imposed external review necessitates nationally-imposed restrictions on management action, which also discourage innovation.

External review based on self-regulation has been claimed to weaken state enforcement and public accountability (The consumer consortium on assisted living newsletter 2000). For example, in the United States, voluntary accreditation is allowed in some states to substitute for formal inspection by state regulatory bodies; this is referred to as deemed status. This is a form of co-regulation in which the achievement of the standards was deemed to meet all necessary quality standards for the purposes of receiving Medicare and Medicaid financing. However, the origins of the standards in a self-regulatory model led to concerns that this form of co-regulation could weaken both state enforcement and public accountability.

In July 1999, the Office of the Inspector General (OIG), which exists to protect the integrity of the Department of Health and Human Services, observed that, contrary to the arguments put forward by the hospital industry in the USA, reliance could not be placed on Joint Commission on Accreditation of Healthcare Organisations (JCAHO) assessments as the surveys, in their opinion, were unlikely to detect substandard patterns of care.

The Office of the Inspector General criticized the JCAHO for relying on a 'collegial' mode of oversight 'which may undermine . . . patient protections'. Furthermore, the Health Care Financing Administration (HCFA) (later retitled (CMS) Center for Medicare and Medicaid Services) 'does little [to hold JCAHO] accountable for their performance'. The report stated that 'HCFA's feedback to the Joint Commission is negligible . . . Indeed, HCFA's posture to the Joint Commission is more deferential than directive' (Office of the Inspector General 1999). The Office of the Inspector General concluded that deemed status 'should not be for perpetuity, without accountability for performance'. That is, the process of external review needs to be rigorously monitored to ensure it is capable of providing adequate assurance to deliver accountability.

Inspection

Inspection based on checking compliance with national standards alone can never deliver the requirements of the new form of governance required by health care systems in which management is devolved and organizations are required to work as networks to provide services.

> Box ticking . . . can be seized upon as the easier option than the diligent pursuit of corporate governance objectives. It would then not be difficult for lazy or unscrupulous directors to arrange matters so that the letter of every governance rule was complied with but not the substance. It might even be possible for the next disaster to emerge in a company, with on paper a 100% record of compliance . . . The true safeguard for good corporate governance lies in the application of informed or independent judgement by experienced and qualified individuals – executive and non-executive directors, shareholders and auditors.
>
> (Hampel Committee report 1998; Mackay and Sweeting 2000)

Furthermore, inspection based on other approaches to assessing quality has also been demonstrated to be flawed and rarely provides adequate levels of assurance. Day and Klein (2004), in their examination of the work of the Commission for Health Improvement (CHI) found that the conceptual framework used for inspection was too focused on a taxonomy of quality rather than on an understanding of what they termed 'the underlying "dynamics" of high quality organisations' (Day and Klein 2004). CHI was accused of failing to know how to examine aspects of good organization, such as culture and leadership. The inspectors were accused of attempting to convert a 'rag-bag of reflections into global and quantified assessments' (Day and Klein 2004).

In addition, regulation through inspection implies a sense of mistrust and, therefore, external controls and external review become unacceptable. This suggests that, instead, a system has to be devised that encourages boards to be able to do their best and to submit their performance to external assessment. According to present theories, this would lead to assessment by stakeholders. But this begs the question, on what basis should judgements be made in this complex world? Although formal controls implemented properly can increase trust, because objective rules and clear measures help to institute a 'track record' for people who do their jobs well (Sitkin and Roth 1993), this is considered to be the major factor contributing to the stifling of the willingness to take risks and the consequent reduction in innovation. The solution, it is argued, must lie in the better internal management of organizations and an improved understanding of internal control, including the creation of a culture which continuously aims to deliver effective and improved services. It is not possible to rely solely on formal external controls but equally society can no longer rely wholly on professional, internal, social controls, which depend upon shared norms and goals. As pointed out in Chapter 1, internal agreement on goals can conflict with public assumptions about the appropriate role and functioning of public services, particularly health services. The arguments, therefore, lead to the view that there is a need for a coherent system of controls which can be externally validated in order to produce assurances that will meet the requirements of the public.

Such a coherent system of controls has to perform three necessary functions if it is to provide adequate accountability. First, the approach must ensure that true but appropriately-designed, independent verification can occur. Second, the approach must not deter innovation and, therefore, must encourage the management of risks. And third, it must provide adequate information to hold the organization to account (Lord Sharman 2002 recommendation 17).

In designing such an approach, it must also be remembered that it has become unacceptable to place a heavy burden of inspection and audit upon health services, as it is held that the impact is neither cost-effective nor useful. Instead, there is a need to replace existing regulation with what has been termed strategic regulation, which focuses on those organizations and services that are at highest risk of failure (Audit Commission 2003). In health care as elsewhere, central government has tended to favour the imposition of performance measures based on the 'general principle of good management that it is usually more effective to define outcomes and objectives rather than to specify precisely how tasks should be carried out' (Performance and Innovation Unit 2001a para 4.6). This is the argument behind the introduction of Public Service Agreements (Performance and Innovation Unit 2001a para 4.7). However, there remains a nervousness in depending wholly on outcome measures to assess performance.

There are, however, cases in which the centre of government will feel justified in doing more than defining the ends that public services should be seeking to achieve. There may be cases where there would be legitimate public concern about variation in services, or where there is clearly established evidence that one approach is the best means of achieving certain ends. In these cases, central government clearly can have a role in defining means as well as ends.

(Performance and Innovation Unit 2001c para 4.9)

An approach, known as lighter touch inspection, has been suggested as the compromise to meet the concerns for less intrusive inspection while retaining a degree of control over processes. In lighter touch inspection is it envisaged that the level of inspection and audit should be proportionate to the assessed performance of authorities, which would allow differential levels of inspection depending upon the performance of the organization. This would enable lighter touch inspection to reduce the burden of inspection for high-performing authorities (Office of the Deputy Prime Minister 2003). However, although this may deliver incentives for innovation and modernization, it leaves a gap in accountability. It does not provide the necessary monitoring to ensure the public is informed that all organizations are delivering the right services in the right way. Lighter touch inspection follows a decision about the level of performance, and does not of itself reveal whether organisations are making decisions well, at the level of the board or the individual practitioner. As long as nothing untoward is noticed, inspections will not be carried out.

The arguments about equity of service delivery, which dominate discussions of health care, lead to concerns about allowing widespread local innovation in clinical practice because of the lack of clear evidence about what works (Performance and Innovation Unit 2001a para 4.11). This conflicts directly with the concepts of modernization and the need for innovation to improve service delivery. In addition, however, there are arguments against too much freedom for local organizations because of the difficulties that arise in what is called the agency relationship.

Agency theory is concerned with the costs of resolving conflicts between the principals (in private companies this is the shareholders) and the agents (in this case the managers), and aligning the interests of the two groups. Agency theory explains how to best organize relationships in which one party (the principal) determines the work, which another party (the agent) undertakes (Eisenhardt 1985). The theory argues that under conditions of incomplete information and uncertainty, which characterize most business settings, two problems arise, known as adverse selection and moral hazard. Adverse selection is the condition under which the principal cannot ascertain if the agent accurately represents his ability to do the work for which he is being paid. Moral hazard is the condition under which the principal cannot be sure if the agent has put forth maximal effort (Eisenhardt 1985). In health care where outputs are so difficult to specify and measure precisely, there is a perceived need for governments to try to control, or at least measure, all the activities of organizations for which they are held responsible.

However, when the focus of accountability shifts towards quality, it is claimed that precise performance measurement is not possible and will not deliver the necessary assurances required by today's public (Donabedian 1980). The purpose of any assessment regarding quality is to pass judgement on the quality of health care, regardless of whether the care was provided by practitioners or institutions, implemented by patients or used by the community. And this requires recognition that 'the concept of quality is itself in large measure a social construct. It represents our conceptions and valuations of health, our expectations of the client-provider relationship and our views of the legitimate roles of the health care enterprise' (Donabedian 1988a page 190). The methods used for the assessment of quality require a degree of negotiation at the local level as well as within a national framework.

Simply producing more information for public consumption also will not achieve greater accountability or assurance. As the previous chapter demonstrated, improved trust and accountability must be built on improved assurance. This leads to the conclusion that what is needed is a different way in which organizations and their managers explain the management of their businesses. O'Neill has referred to this as intelligent accountability based on principles of good governance. 'Serious and effective accountability needs to concentrate on good governance, on obligations to tell the truth and needs to seek intelligent accountability' (O'Neill 2002). Obligation to tell the truth is important. Infrequently, but regularly, cases are brought to light in which organizations and their managers are accused of cheating, or gaming the performance management system. Indicators of the size of waiting lists, for example, are found to have been altered to reveal a better picture than really exists. The incentives to game with statistical indicators are many, and although the sanctions are often harsh for cheating, the risks of making fraudulent returns are considered worth taking, especially when the sanctions attached to honest reporting indicate failure to achieve the required levels of performance is equivalent to cheating. There is a need to build incentives that promote a need to declare the risks of failure and the opportunity to demonstrate how those risks will be managed in the future.

Intelligent accountability and Statements of Internal Control

Intelligent accountability focuses on good governance of public organizations but it recognizes that accountability cannot be sustained on the basis of 'informal relations of trust'. O'Neill argues that conditions of trust are only feasible where individuals can check the information provided by others.

Organizations and their managers need to be encouraged to disclose where there are systemic failures, which create the strategic risks that lead to the inability to achieve performance targets and strategic objectives. The Statement on Internal Control provides the opportunity for a range of disclosures, which include both identifying failures in the management system and the associated remedies being put in place. This encourages the production of better public information, which will permit public scrutiny of the actions of managers which, in turn, encourages managers to be honest about the workings of the health care system for which they are responsible, as well as providing an opportunity to disclose the reasons for failure to succeed. Decision-making processes need to be exposed to public scrutiny in a way that allows the public and politicians to understand and judge the quality of the management decisions made. Judgements need to be made on the basis of a balance between expert and public opinion on the nature and the scale of the risk faced and how well it was managed (Cabinet Office 2002).

To reconstitute existing approaches to the regulation of health care without recognizing the centrality of the complex dimensions of quality will not deliver acceptable accountability. In addition, if the approach does not tackle the fundamental issue of how to increase trust while also encouraging a desire to improve, it will not produce the required devolved management and desired local public accountability. It is imperative that the emergent system of regulation recognizes the need to encourage health care organizations to take responsibility for the improvement of quality of care and to demonstrate that they are succeeding in doing this. What is required is the public sector health care equivalent of what Tricker describes as being needed in the private sector: 'a vibrant alternative way to ensure that power is exercised, over every type and form of corporate entity and strategic alliance . . . in a way that ensures both effective performance and appropriate social accountability and responsibility' (Tricker 1994).

One solution offered to encourage greater organizational responsibility for quality of health care has been to place the responsibility for management and accountability on the shoulders of individual board-level directors.

> At the level of individual trusts, an executive member of the board should have the responsibility for putting into operation the trust's strategy and policy on safety in clinical care. Further, a non-executive director should be given specific responsibility for providing leadership to the strategy and policy aimed at securing safety in clinical care.
> (The Report of the Public Inquiry into children's heart surgery at the Bristol Royal Infirmary 1984–1995 2001 para 121)

But this places the responsibility of running separate parts of what should be an integrated organizational structure on individual directors. Furthermore, given the complexity of health care organizations, it is probably too much to ask of individual directors. Board level responsibility for the actions of the organization and its performance should be shared and the board held equally accountable to the public they serve.

Good governance, in both the private and public sectors, is equated with internal control through risk management in order to achieve objectives. But such decisions about the management of risks and their associated controls have to be independently validated and made visible (Power 1997). As discussed above, the experience of inspection and audit has demonstrated that they focus too readily on the eradication of risk, and management have tended to follow the lead of their auditors. This has led not only to the stifling of the willingness of staff to innovate, but also to the stifling of the desire to improve quality of services. As Donabedian (1988b) has pointed out, attempts to reduce error to zero creates additional cost, which is not commensurate with the increase in the quality of service. A new approach to accountability requires a formal process of assurance based on the value and substance of decisions and actions taken to tackle risks to the public, the services and the finances of the organization. The future lies in the development of better risk management, a better understanding of internal control systems and appropriate methods for auditing them.

The developments in the private sector demonstrated that boards should focus their attention on the strategic risks, that is those relevant to the achievement of objectives, rather than operational risks. For the NHS to be accountable as a single organization, it is necessary to have a system that demonstrates the management of risks not only on a local level but also against national performance targets. This requires that there is a single system which sets national objectives and can assess risks to achieving them at every level of the NHS, through to the Department of Health.

It has been suggested frequently that the NHS should be freed from political control by the introduction of an independent central management function, for example, an NHS Corporation which would allow the government to set the strategic direction for the NHS but leave performance management and assuring accountability to the NHS (Dewar 2003; King's Fund 2002). The benefits of such a body would be to replicate what is already undertaken under the NHS, while removing the setting of national standards and targets from the personalities of politicians and the preferences of political parties. But to some extent these must be determined by politicians acting on behalf of their citizens. As discussed earlier, it is no longer possible to accept that the definition of quality in terms of care, access or treatment lies solely within the province of professional or health service employees. Merely transferring control from the Department of Health to another central body would not increase the devolution of decision making which is required to improve public accountability.

The single set of clear objectives also needs to enshrine a single approach to the definition of quality. This is for two reasons. One is to provide a framework that provides a consistency for the definition of good quality, which can be used to ensure the uniformity of approaches to quality across the national health service. There must be a structure which provides incentives and motivation to ensure that decisions are carried out (Spangenberg 2001). If managers and clinicians are rational human beings, they will only work towards the same objectives if they share them. The second reason, important in a system of devolved management, is to offer a degree of protection to the people within the health care system charged with commissioning and designing health care. In a case in the USA an HMO was sued by a patient who received poor care and subsequently died. The HMO responded that it had done its best – it had, on behalf of the employer who provided the insurance cover for the patient, contracted with a provider who would provide services of an acceptable quality. However, the judges' conclusion was somewhat different in that while there was no doubt in their minds that all concerned expected the medical services arranged by the HMO to be of acceptable quality, this seemed to them to be beside the point. 'The relevant inquiry is not whether there was an expectation of acceptably competent services but rather whether there was an agreement to displace the quality standard found in otherwise applicable law with a contract standard' (Rosenbaum and Teitelbaum 2000). That is, it was felt that the HMO had used its own assessment of quality in deciding what was acceptable for the provider to provide and, in so doing, had made its own decisions about the definition of quality. For this it was held to be responsible. One interpretation of this finding could be that without national standards, Primary Care Trusts and other purchasing organizations would be vulnerable as a result of applying their own definitions of quality.

Systems of accountability

Accountability, particularly in public services, cannot leave governance entirely to the board of directors, interested groups and the auditors. The general public also has an interest in the running of public services and accountability and as described earlier, requires assurances that the public good is not being put at risk. The trust in public service managers and clinicians is no longer strong enough to sustain these informal relationships. Governance itself is changing to address how organizations communicate values and choices to the public and users, and promote accountability for good as well as poor performance (Audit Commission 2003) – including the ability for users to raise concerns if they are not satisfied with services (National Audit Office 2001a para 21). There is still a need for some form of independent external review, which will provide the necessary public assurance but which will not impose unnecessary bureaucracy and central prescription through dictat.

Trust and accountability also require that health care services deliver what the public expects of them. This necessitates some form of performance measurement against collected statistics. Internal controls will generate internal performance management.

> In a well designed system or institution, much information about performance is obtained informally or incidentally by collaborative work, discussion, consultation, conferences and the like. Whatever can be done to ... make the work of colleagues visible to each other, creates an incentive for each one to perform at a level that at least avoids embarrassment and certainly censure. But there is also a need for a specific organisational unit whose primary function is to monitor clinical performance continuously, impartially and consistently.
>
> (Donabedian 1989 page 6)

Local stakeholder management of performance carried out continuously, impartially and consistently will contribute to local accountability, but in a national health service there will doubtless continue to be a requirement for national stakeholders to have some representation in the accountability structure. It would appear this can only be achieved through the design of a performance management system that creates a system of formal control over the total system, including decision making, service specification, and the mechanisms used to reward or sanction current behaviour designed to influence future behaviour. This formal control is frequently conducted using measures and targets to assess objectively the performance of an organization, thereby leading to improved future performance and reinforcing accountability (Lord Sharman 2002). There is a need, therefore, for a governance and accountability system which combines the three key elements of public sector control – external control, internal control and performance management – into a single system of accountability designed to promote devolved management (see figure 7.1).

For there to be a National Health Service, rather than a set of wholly independent organizations, there needs to be an overarching national strategy that provides key objectives for all NHS organizations. These objectives must be stated in ways that provide a national structure for the internal control of the day-to-day operations of health care, which can only be described in terms of processes and the assessment of outcomes, that is, performance. There also needs to be a recognition that operational systems and performance management must be designed to act synergistically – they must support each other. This must underpin the framework for providing assurance to the public that the health service is designed to deliver the outcomes they want and to manage the risks that they wish it to manage. The design of the operating system requires the development of national standards, a solution which the

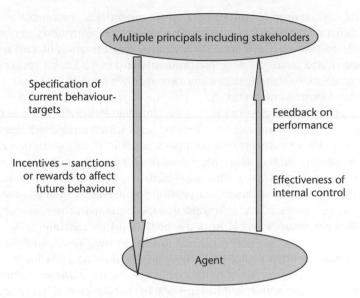

Figure 7.1 The accountability system.

government has espoused for many years. The design of the performance monitoring system must provide assurance against measures that reflect these standards. But the focus of the review systems must be upon risk management, and auditors must learn to deal with the assessment of risk. Even where risk taking has featured as the focus of audit, auditors have still been perceived as discouraging well-managed risk taking. Auditors have been urged to ensure that their work lives up to the spirit of statements made on attitudes to innovation (Lord Sharman 2002).

New governance

The principles underpinning new governance demand that boards are left free to establish coherent systems of internal control and they must demonstrate that these systems are effective to manage risks. Risk management in this context has two functions. One is to establish that decisions within the organization, from the board and elsewhere, were not taken in ways that put the organization or patients, staff and other users at risk, and the other is that the national objectives were achieved. In addition, new governance assumes that boards will be required to make a public declaration that they understand their objectives (both performance and operational) and that they are managing their organizations so as to achieve them. The Statement on Internal Control is the public declaration by the board that it can provide reasonable assurance that it has taken these objectives into account. Organizations also need to demonstrate that they are actually achieving performance in line with the operational and strategic objectives and this is done through a streamlined performance management system, which also allows risks to be escalated to the central Department of Health.

The model of new governance for the National Health Service has to combine into a single coherent whole all the features which any government of the day has laid out in various different places. That is, there has to be a balance between regulation, auditable internal control systems, professional control systems and social control within organizations. The balance has to be set by the centre so that boards and organizations understand what is expected of them, and the public is able to engage in a dialogue with their local organizations, in order to understand how the board and its staff are to be held to account. However, these controls must not be overly prescriptive. To permit devolved management to flourish, they must be fluid and flexible enough to permit local diversity while working within a standard framework. They must encourage and support the development of networks and alliances while ensuring that organizations can be held appropriately accountable. They must encourage focus on the needs and care of individual patients, while recognising the need for local priorities to be determined locally.

According to the theory of internal control, there must be a central identification of a single set of objectives and the strategic risks to achieving them, which provides the cohesion needed to ensure all the independent components of the NHS work together to achieve a set of agreed aims, to ensure each citizen receives the same quality of health care. However, most of the risk management ability of the NHS, through the structure of controls assurance, had focused on dealing with operational risks such as health and safety. The command and control structure of the NHS, developed through an overly bureaucratic performance management regime devised around output controls, had led NHS boards to focus on the achievement of targets rather than the development of rigorous risk management. NHS boards, therefore, tended to develop two independent strategic management processes, one focusing on achieving performance targets and the other focusing on operational risk management.

New governance requires that there is a single system of risk management, which integrates and compares top-down strategic risks management processes with bottom-up control and risk assessment approaches (Standards Australia 2000). In health care, systems theory is central to the current understanding of quality and provides the needed link between the elements of quality and control. Systems theory presents the opportunity to marry the top-down, strategic approaches to achieving risk objectives with the bottom-up approach of identifying those operational risks which may jeopardize integrity and survival of the organization. The operating systems are the elements which both create and are shaped by the culture of the organization and enable it to reduce hazards in the care of patients.

> Current conceptual thinking on the safety of patients places prime responsibility for adverse events on deficiencies in system design, organisation and operation rather than on individual providers or individual products . . . Most adverse events are not the result of neg-ligence or lack of training but rather occur because of latent causes within systems . . . For those who work on systems, adverse events are shaped and provoked by 'upstream' systemic factors, which include the particular organisation's strategy, its culture, its approach towards quality management and risk prevention and its capacity for learning from failures. Counter measures based on changes in the system are therefore more productive than those that target individual practices or products.
>
> (World Health Organisation Secretariat 2001 page 2)

It is probably fair to say that in the early days of the introduction of the Statement on Internal Control (SIC), signed by all chief executives on behalf of their boards, it was rarely perceived by NHS boards as a document describing the effective control of risks to the government's strategic objectives, nor as indication of the achievement of the performance based output controls. Instead, the Statement on Internal Control was seen as a declaration of con-trols relating to operational areas. It was possible for boards to act as though there was a discontinuity between the top-down and bottom-up assessments of risk within the Statement of Internal Control, which meant that, as an assurance tool, the Statement on Internal Control was only partially effective and did not provide evidence of an organization-wide approach to control. The limited impact of the Statement on Internal Control was partly due to the slow process of its introduction and the slow understanding of how internal control should be used for accountability purposes within government departments and subsequently applied to the NHS. The Treasury identified the need for the SIC to refer to 'significant internal control problems'. Although it was explained that this phrase could not be absolutely defined because signifi-cance depended on circumstances; one example of a significant internal control problem was that 'it prejudices the achievement of a Public Service Agreement target'. When the guidance from the Treasury was translated into the requirements placed on the NHS, the explanation no longer referred to Public Service Agreement targets. Instead, NHS organizations were advised to consider whether the issue seriously prejudiced or prevented achievement of a principal objective.

A key issue in considering the accountability arrangements for the NHS is whether NHS organizations can be expected to mature to a point at which the focus of risk management is on strategic risk, as suggested by the Cabinet Office, or whether there has to continue to be a detailed requirement to demonstrate the management of operational risks and hazards because these are such an important and integral part of the delivery of safe health care. Advice provided from central government on how to focus NHS board attention on particular risks has varied. The Turnbull report had recommended the board focus on ten risks, but the advice on implementing Turnbull suggested fifteen to twenty-five (Centre for Business Performance 1999) – although some firms were reported as having identified many more (Deloitte and Touche 2000). The advice developed for government departments suggested that boards should identify a limited number, ten to fifteen high-level risks or those associated with organizational strategy, which can be considered and managed by senior management, in order to increase the organization's ability to meet its objectives. The Department of Health, in contrast, advised NHS boards that they should handle 75 to 200 risks and the board's assurance committees would give priority to reporting routinely the current top six to twelve risk issues to the Board (Department of Health 2002a). The Department of Health felt that the board should be aware of operational risks because of the need to protect patients and staff from hazards – and this demonstrates the difficulties faced by NHS boards. The advice supplied on the implementation of the Turnbull recommendations suggested a top-down approach, in order to focus attention only on strategic significant risks (Deloitte and Touche 2000). The risks generated by assurance committees, which were derived from organizational risk registers, would inevitably reflect operational risks, thus preventing the integration of operational risks with the risks to achieving strategic objectives. Boards tended to replace considerations of strategic objectives with concerns about the targets required by the separate performance management processes of central government, which frequently generated a conflict with local operating objectives such as safety.

The result was that boards frequently received information on the achievement of targets in isolation from the deliberations of their committees which examined issues, such as patient safety. In a number of cases, this was because it was easier and less contentious for boards to isolate the activities rather than see them as part of the same exercise. When a target was produced which required the reduction of waiting times, hospitals tended to ignore safety or service delivery considerations, such as appropriate staffing levels, in favour of achieving the waiting time requirements. This resulted in the organization being forced into carrying risks which it would not itself have chosen to accept. Too many risks can lead to information overload, the number of the nature of risks that the board and the individuals within the organization can cope with needs to be well understood (Centre for Business Performance 1999 page 9). 'Cumbersome risk management databases can be a distraction from the key point which is that each person in the organisation becomes more focused on meeting business objectives and in managing significant risks which relate to the tasks which he or she performs' (The Internal Control Working Party of the Institute of Chartered Accountants in England and Wales 1999).

A new approach to assurance

Although a system of devolved management, such as that sought for the NHS, requires individual organizations to take responsibility for identifying and managing their risks through a system of control within their own organizations, these organizations remain part of a single National Health Service. The ideas of holistic governance mentioned above argue for a new form of accountability, in which organizations are held to account for their contribution to key objectives (Perry 6 1997). This can produce a justification of the actions taken but does not address issues of procedural probity or equity. The recently emerging ideas of governance require that instead of outcome-based or target-based performance management, there should be a nationally agreed process of continuous review of the identification, assessment and management of risk in achieving nationally agreed, strategic objectives for health care.

This confirms the need for a single standardized framework for internal control, in order to allow the Chief Executive of the NHS to declare that controls across the NHS are effective in producing care that cuts across organizational boundaries. However, the dependence of health care upon teams of professionals means that such a standardized system would have to encompass not only hard controls but also the softer controls deriving from the practice of medicine. In any organization of people, the essence of control is purpose, commitment, monitoring and learning (Criteria of Control Board of the Canadian Institute of Chartered Accountants 1995) and, therefore, the key to control in this form of governance has to be ensuring purpose and commitment rather than any externally-imposed requirements or regulations. Health care organizations are dependent upon professional teams, acting in concert to deliver modern health. For two reasons, their professionalism and their team membership, they have to be trusted to perform their tasks appropriately. This means, in turn, that the internal control system has to recognize that the degree to which any societal system achieves its set objectives will depend upon the attention placed on those norms, rules and elements which shape behaviours and which will focus behaviour on objectives (Eisenhardt 1985). The framework, therefore, needs to based upon an understanding of how to achieve an appropriate balance between different types of controls.

Sophisticated approaches to assessment are required, which need to include the factors influencing the organizational perception of risk and also an accepted definition of what is reasonable assurance. NHS boards need to recognize the implications of signing a statement declaring they have done all they could do to meet their objectives and ensure the safety and welfare of their staff, patients and others. Boards and their organizations must steer their way through a complex and difficult strategic management task of assuring public accountability through a welter of legislative requirements, without losing the focus on their primary task of promoting health and providing health care. Boards also need to understand how these decisions need to be made in conjunction with their main stakeholders, including their publics, to ensure that decisions meet with the requirements of public accountability. This requires organizations to educate their publics in the issues concerning the risks on which they have to take decisions, and to ensure their risk taking is in line with the public evaluation of risk. But this will necessitate continuous public involvement as the subjective nature of risk suggests that perceptions of risk change with time and external circumstances. Risks in public policy, which require the accommodation of many different perceptions, are treated in a similar way to that described by Braybrooke and Lindblom four decades ago as synthetic:

> For a cluster of interlocked problems can always be formally envis-
> aged as one problem, in which 'the problem' is to find a reconciliation
> of the diverse groups on terms that provide a measure of satisfaction
> for each ... Problem solving becomes a more continuous process
> than is ordinarily thought. Whether or not a possible reconciliation
> today is satisfactory will depend on what yesterday's pattern of
> reconciliation was and what tomorrow's might be.
>
> (Braybrooke and Lindblom 1963 page 55)

Within the nationally agreed framework, according to the control literature, boards will need to establish values and cultures that encourage individuals to focus on risks, and encourage boards and management to find
incentives to motivate personnel not only to manage risks but also to take
them appropriately. However, management in this context has to be appropriate and provide the right incentives, if it is not to create devastating
unanticipated consequences. If controls have a negative effect on individual
motivation, or reduce the interest of the individual in organizational goals,
they could increase the chance of risky decisions being taken (Walsh and
Schneider 2002).

> Boards appear to take inadequate steps to secure successful policy
> implementation and remain unclear about and ambivalent toward
> matters of accountability ... The fundamental problem in terms
> of corporate performance resides in the fact that the majority of

directors (Chairs excepted) are unclear about their statutory obligations and legal responsibilities. . . . The lack of clarity which seems
to bedevil Non-executive directors creates tensions and boundary
disputes between themselves and executive directors.

(Harrison 1998 page 147)

The board's role, therefore, is to provide active leadership, within a nationally
recognized framework of prudent and effective controls, which enable risk to
assessed and managed (Appointments Commission & Department of Health
2003 page 9). Boards have to develop rigorous approaches to evaluating the
adequacy of their organization's risk and control framework and must check
that the framework is able to respond to a rapidly changing environment.
They must also ensure that they are not placing too great an assurance burden
on the organization. The board has to ensure proportionality of control so that
it does not stifle the workings of the organization. (HM Treasury 2000b para
7.4). But for this to provide a socially acceptable level of assurance, there must
be a corresponding acceptance on the part of the public served that assurance
is not absolute. Proportional control can only provide reasonable assurance
not perfect assurance.

For assurance to work in this way, it is necessary that the public, whether
as tax payers or patients, understand the risks that the board is managing on
their behalf. Not all risks can be foreseen but the board is responsible for ensuring that adequate controls are in place to manage foreseeable risks. Reasonable
assurance is only possible when all parties, including all stakeholders, understand what is reasonable to expect of a board or its employees. Communication with the public and adequate consultation is, therefore, vitally important.

Boards have to accept that they are responsible for explaining to the public what they believe they have control over and must disclose risks they have
identified but feel they do not have under control, if public accountability is to
be achieved. Few private businesses were willing and able to implement the
Turnbull recommendations when they were introduced. An increasing body of
evidence has demonstrated that boards of directors failed to understand their
responsibilities in this area and, as a consequence were not involved in properly managing their companies (Finkelstein and Hambrick 1996 page 228).
Boards were more likely to be involved in ratifying strategies presented to
them by senior managers and were unlikely to challenge powerful Chief
Executives (Finkelstein and Hambrick 1996 page 171).

Our concern is not so much with extraordinary circumstances but
with the ongoing process of governance where independent directors
of a controlled company may have difficulties from time to time in
carrying out what we have described as the core functions of governance. Particularly important, in our view, are the selection of (and

ability, where appropriate, to terminate) the CEO and a meaningful
involvement in developing the strategic direction of the company. If
the board of a controlled corporate is not playing a meaningful role in
these functions, then it appears to us that it is more in the nature of
an advisory board than a board of directors.

(Final report Joint Committee on Corporate Governance 2001
page 25)

Health care also requires that controls focus on quality of service delivery
and the board has to ensure that it establishes controls which can deliver
continuous quality improvement, rather than just box-ticking quality assurance. Quality improvement is substantively different from quality assurance
when considered in an agency framework.

Using the agency framework, three substantive differences are noted
when comparing the board's role in quality improvement relative to
quality assurance. First, under quality improvement relative emphasis
on social, behaviour and outcome controls employed by the board
shifts to place greater importance on social control. Second, agency
accountabilities are defined to focus less on individual managers or
physicians and more on collectivities of individuals comprising systems or processes that contribute to quality of care. Finally the scope
of the board's activity under quality improvement is expanded
beyond the narrow parameters of externally mandated programmes
such as quality assurance into a broader array of internal and external
functions.

(Weiner and Alexander 1993 page 389)

In this analysis, the principal control strategy for quality improvement is
social control. Boards need to align the preferences of their agents (professional staff) with those of their principals (their stakeholders) by fostering a
common set of values concerning the importance of continuous improvement. Boards need to do this through a variety of social control mechanisms,
which Weiner and Alexander identify as intensive selection, training and
socialization. 'Social control enables boards to shift the focus of control in
quality improvement from outcomes attributable to individual agents to performance and capability of production processes' (Weiner and Alexander 1993
Page 390). This is tantamount to saying that the agent is no longer defined as
an individual manager or physician but a system or set of processes that
embrace multiple individuals in collective endeavour. Such a focus is consistent with the quality improvement proposition that individual performance is
the result of a complex interaction of people and support systems (Deming
2002). Moreover, since responsibility for exerting control over a production

process rests with process owners, the focus of board activities in quality improvement shifts from exercising control over agents to creating an institutional context that fosters quality leadership, sustains constancy of purpose with respect to quality improvement, and removes organizational barriers to continuous improvement. Again, clinical governance was introduced to deliver precisely this focus on continuous quality improvement in clinical professional practice (Scally and Donaldson 1998).

Accountability and networks

A new approach to governance and accountability has to recognize that the structures of health care organizations are changing. No longer can health care be provided in single hierarchical structures. Instead, these are being replaced by interconnected organizations, such as networks and partnerships, better suited, it is hoped, to meet the complex needs of individual citizens. The term 'holistic governance' has been coined to describe the new form of governance required for organizations that collaborate to provide services (Perry 6 1997) and requires that networks approach this by first defining the goals of collaboration and then designing services and interventions to deliver them. Within the European Union, new governance has begun to appear as a new approach to central regulation. There is a move from top-down, uniform rules using top-down command and control regulation backed by sanctions (hard laws) to a more flexible and participatory approach, which has been referred to as 'soft law' (Trubeck and Mosher 2001). These new governance arrangements have been called 'the open-method of co-ordination' (Trubeck and Mosher 2001 page 1). New governance also has to focus on how to create co-ordination and co-operation across networks of many organizations, to ensure 'joined-up' accountability, as well as dealing with individual organizations (National Audit Office 2001a).

Governance in health care networks is a complex issue, particularly if patients are to be accorded individual care designed and tailored to their needs. A wide range of organizations need to be brought together to meet the needs of some highly-dependent groups, such as the elderly infirm, those with chronic conditions or the mentally ill. In private sector organizations, a network or association of firms may itself be considered as a firm or as an organizational whole (Richter 1994 page 24). Networks of firms come together in an architecture which is frequently similar in behaviour to that of individual firms in that a network of information processing and control centres is required to make the structure function. There is frequently a unitary board, which sits above the network to control it and can be treated like similar entities in single firms in which investment risks of related parties can be modified by ownership and control structures and where the board shares and manages risk (Hart and Moore 1990).

Unlike private sector networks, which mostly exist on an intra-firm basis, public sector networks are inter-organizational structures with a number of independent boards, which do not work together to share risk or investment opportunities. Therefore, these public sector networks are not established structures but are loose confederations of service delivery organizations, such as departments, agencies and voluntary and private sector organizations, which undertake joint working to provide complementary services. For these services to work together there needs to be co-ordination which, if poorly managed, puts at risk the whole system of service delivery. 'For example, if part of the service provided by one organisation is delayed or is of poor quality the success of the whole programme is put at risk' (Public Accounts Committee 2001 para 17). Relationships and lines of responsibility become more complicated in these structures (Performance and Innovation Unit 2000; (Lord Sharman 2002). The distance of the services from central government gives rise to complex delivery chains, involving many different organizations, which makes it impossible to devise a single coherent structure and increases the risk that improvements in public services take a long time to achieve (National Audit Office 2004).

The recommended solution is that organizations must find ways to assess the risk management of partner organisations and that clear accountability for risks is identified (Cabinet Office 2002 4.3.34). For example, the complex pattern of organizations involved in service delivery was felt to have contributed to a lack of clear accountability in the case of railway accidents in the UK. The recommendation was clearer lines of accountability to central government departments who could monitor performance and take appropriate action. 'We recommend that where responsibility for risk is transferred to a partner organisation, particular care is taken to ensure that accountabilities are clearly established by Departments, procedures for escalating risks are agreed, and capacity maintained to manage and monitor performance (including provision of relevant information) and to take early action in the event of difficulty' (Cabinet Office 2002). The Public Accounts Committee recommended the use of a national risk management standard as the basis for accrediting partners' risk management arrangements (Public Accounts Committee 2001 para 17).

This approach to risk suggests that the management of risk is still contained within individual organizations, in that one organisation should monitor the risk approaches of other organizations. This is not the same as developing an integrated approach to risk management for those services that require integration from the patient perspective. The Audit Commission has also recently drawn attention to the need for an approach to risk management which can accommodate different organizations working together.

Governance in networks is complicated because professionals need to operate through horizontal relationships, which enable the creation of adhocracies, teams brought together to provide care to individual patients. There has been much discussion in the literature on the appropriate methods for maintaining accountability for professional action. Where professional accountability structures are kept separate from management accountability structures, there have been concerns about professionals using limited resources in ways that do not achieve the strategic objectives of the organization. Placing professionals under the direct management of lay general managers was not felt to provide adequate professional support, a basic requirement of professional people. An alternative approach was to use what was termed 'matrix management', in which professionals worked to two separate lines of accountability, one for general management and resource purposes and another relating to professional decision making and actions. Matrix management rarely worked well as it led to confusion and split accountability and, therefore, was abandoned in favour of direct line management provided by professionals by placing professionals in corporate management units, such as clinical directorates. A clinical director would head the management structure, and be responsible for a budget and for the actions taken within the unit.

The discussion on the correct way to manage professionals continues, and presents issues for the consideration of the development of controls and the provision of assurance and accountability.

> We think there should be different lines of accountability for matters of professional competence and for matters of day-to-day management. We think the profession itself is best placed to lead on matters of professional competence. This is because professional input will always be required when specialist technical issues arise. This does not mean we oppose proper checks and balances to ensure that the system operates in the public interest. These are vital. We also think that the employer, or body that is contracting with doctors for services (which may complicate the situation for controlling the behaviour of GPs) has a duty to set out and enforce adequate controls over a doctor's duties under contract. This would include the NHS (as employer) establishing systems that allow it to be certain of the professional competence of those it is managing.
>
> (Better regulation task force 2000a para 4.4.2.2).

The interesting feature about a network that works across organizational boundaries is that it requires a different approach to governance. Professionals tend to be employed to work within existing organizational structures, which have their own boards and, therefore, their own governance arrangements. When profesionals work within a network, which takes their work outside their own organization, there is no formal governance of their activities within the network. The controls which are in place are designed to operate solely within the organization that employs them.

Furthermore, alliances or partnerships suffer from low output measurability; that is, it is difficult to assess their outcome (Das and Teng 2001). The risks in partnerships are referred to as relational risks, they derive from the problems that occur when one organisation and its employees with one culture works closely with another. The actions of one organization impact upon another. Relational risk derives from the possibility of poor co-operation between organizations. Simply being aware of another organization's risks is not enough and neither are output controls. There is a need to use behaviour control mechanisms, such as rules about the exchange of information, to reduce the risks. If output controls, such as performance measures, are to be used, they have to be agreed between the partners and the measure chosen will depend on the bargaining power of the parties involved (Aimin and Gray 1994). This, therefore, requires a co-ordinated approach to developing appropriate controls which recognizes the significance of behavioural controls.

There is a need to develop further the understanding of the differences between professional and managerial accountability, between accountability for delivery of high-quality clinical services and the delivery of good governance. Networks are based upon assumptions of clinical accountability and require strong lines of accountability from one professional to another. These run outside traditional organizational forms, where accountability is placed upon boards. There needs to be a approach to developing these different forms of accountability and a recognition that they must run parallel but support each other to produce the necessary holistic approach required by new governance. Attempts to bring these into one coherent framework will probably be doomed to failure. They must work synergistically to produce an assurance and accountability framework which reflects the correct balance of social and formal controls, capable of management at the local level.

The development of the model of assurance under devolved management suggests that stakeholders, including the general public, need to be invited to help assess the effectiveness of internal controls of organizations and networks, and the nature of the risk management system, as well as the quality and outcome measures against which the local services are judged. This will require local agreement on the strategic objectives for each organization and a general understanding of the risks attached to achieving them and must include financial and other risks, including those concerning patient safety. The logic of this argument leads inexorably to a very wide role for public and patient involvement, closer to an extended membership of the local authority scrutiny committees. This is necessary for the longer term sustainability of public sector organizations in which power is devolved. Hirschman argued that if consumers are prevented from commenting on the quality of services, voices will be engaged 'only when deterioration has reached so advanced a stage that recovery is no longer possible or desirable' (Hirschman 1970 page 121). For voice to work in this model of accountability, it will be necessary to decide how to select representative stakeholders and when to ask for the assessment of the general public. The public is considered to be cynical about being consulted on issues that they feel are the province of public officials, who should be providing quality services (Strategy unit 2002 page 26). Over- consultation can paralyse not only managerial autonomy, but also public participation.

To some extent, this will be seen as an attempt to create a post-modern interpretation of culture in policy.

> A post-modern perspective on organisational culture would not focus on cultures as a means of control. It would instead encourage dialogue on the nature and course of change among stakeholders, particularly those who traditionally have been disenfranchised or marginalized from such discussions. The emphasis of such a dialogue would be on challenging existing authorized accounts and balances or power rather than on the refinement of mechanisms of control.
>
> (Davies, Nutley and Mannion 2000 page 113)

Current policy reflects this interpretation of inclusion and redefinition of control in recognition of the fact that there is no single, universally accepted means of determining the quality of health care. Locally run health services will require locally-determined assessments of how well organizations deliver not only the corporate governance agenda but also the clinical governance agenda.

With clearly-stated, centrally-defined outcome objectives, and the standards which define the parameters of operational quality, there is a need for two separate but inextricably linked assurance processes. One provides limited performance management to the government which is responsible for the health of its citizens, to ensure that the services are delivering what it has promised the public. The other provides the necessary assurance from the board that the internal control systems, formal and informal, are in its assessment thereby providing reasonable assurance. The Healthcare Commission must provide an assessment of the local relationship between the assurance provided by the board on its internal control systems and the management processes that are in place to meet its objectives within the operational framework set by the health care standards and the performance management regime of the Department of Health. This is necessary to achieve the required public accountability.

> At the formal level, accountability needs to be (and is proposed to be) for the processes of managing towards outcomes, rather than the

outcomes themselves. At the informal level, it is likely that improved information about outcomes, strategies and capabilities will influence the views of those with decision and information rights about quality of judgement and performance.

(Anderson and Dovey 2003 page 9)

In this model, inspection needs to focus on internal control without introducing either formal, externally-designed controls or over control. The basis for inspection has to be a method for reviewing the internal quality assurance processes. The Chairman of the new commission, Sir Ian Kennedy, has called for intelligent scrutiny – a concept using language that is in sympathy with the new trend of intelligent accountability and intelligent audit. The commission will need to focus on the issues of internal control and its relationship with the achievement of performance measures and it will need to focus on risk management and the new organizational forms, such as networks. In so doing, it will need to base its work on the concept of new governance and use an improved form of audit, which requires auditors to standardize audit approaches, which in turn will encourage local flexibility and innovation, and will recognize the need to serve the demands for accountability exercised by a wide range of stakeholders. What is needed, therefore, is intelligent audit which can match intelligent accountability (O'Neill 2002).

Intelligent audit

Intelligent audit needs to differ from old style auditing, which was felt to encourage risk averse behaviour in those audited (Lord Sharman 2002), in that it must promote innovation and well managed risk taking in service delivery. The ideas relating to devolved management suggest it will need to take the best of external review procedure to promote good practice and apply encouragement to organisations, while at the same time delivering needed assurance to the public. The logic of devolved management suggests that audit will need to focus on internal controls and internal risk management systems, closely tied to the delivery of clearly-stated organizational objectives, but recognize that there are multiple accountabilities and seek to address these (Scrivens 2004) (see figure 7.2).

Intelligent audit based on these competing aims will have limitations, which must be recognized by the public and politicians. If it focuses on internal control systems (clinical and organizational), absolute assurance cannot be provided. Inevitably, there will be a price to be paid for devolved management and a dependency on internal control (The Canadian Institute of Chartered Accountants 1995 page 3). As explained in Chapter 3, human behaviour can always over-ride formal control systems. The more important

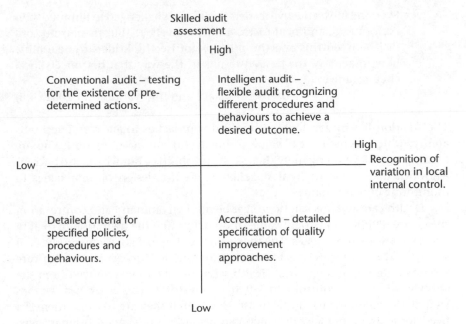

Figure 7.2 Different approaches to external review.

element is getting the appropriate culture and values embedded in the organization and instilling an awareness of risk management at every level. Staff must be permitted to apply intelligent problem solving, to produce the needed innovation, and controls must be limited to those which are necessary to manage significant risks. Intelligent audit must develop to examine how culture, risk management and problem solving are addressed within the organization. It must be grounded in the recognition that costs of control must be balanced against the benefits, including the risks it is designed to manage. This will include choosing forms of audit that will need to be negotiated with local publics, as with all other aspects of performance review and accountability that are outside of a nationally agreed framework. Intelligent accountability will require a considerable amount of trust in intelligent devolved management. If the benefits of devolved management are to be felt, there is a need to allow managers to manage. 'If we want a culture of public service, professionals and public servants must in the end be free to serve the public rather than their paymasters' (O'Neill 2002).

For quality in health care to be delivered, as described in Chapter 1, autonomy of professional staff must be valued highly, as should the ability of the organization as a whole to deliver new and improved services. However, there has to be a mechanism to ensure that freedom at the local level does not become an alternative to accountability.

> Even the most effective leaders need to be challenged to improve their performance and held to account effectively . . . But there is no conflict between this and the principle of freeing leaders to determine how to achieve the desired results in the way that best meets local circumstances.
>
> (Performance and Innovation Unit 2001a 4.8)

The solution lies in developing improved approaches to audit and accountability, which recognize the value of intelligent autonomous staff who are continuously developing individual skills and abilities, but which also encourage open dialogue with local stakeholders in the design of approaches to monitoring of performance.

Health care systems can no longer be run by command and control from the centre. Public and patient values must determine the definition of quality and its assessment processes. The centre, in the shape of government, the civil service and its agencies, has to let go if the public is to get the health care services it desires and requires. Health services have to be removed from the shackles of central control and left to innovate. As this book has demonstrated, the components already exist. However, if they are to work, there is a need for a single framework which can be easily understood by managers, clinicians and the public. The arguments outlined in this book demonstrate that, if the current thinking to achieve improved quality and accountability through increasingly devolved management is implemented, there will have to be further consideration of stakeholder involvement, developments in the understanding of the governance of networks and partnership working, and a commitment to innovation and continuous improvement. And more importantly, new approaches to audit and inspection will be needed, focused upon ways to improve the level of trust the public have in the services established for their benefit.

Chapter Summary

This chapter has dealt with the following points:
- Maintaining accountability when power is devolved through self-regulation, inspection, intelligent accountability, Statements of Internal Control and an accountability system.
- The implementation of new governance in the NHS, the new approach to assurance that this has necessitated.
- The problems of maintaining accountability when working in networks or partnerships.
- The use of intelligent auditing to identify and control risk and deliver quality.

References

Aimin, Y. and Gray, B. (1994) Bargaining power, management control, and performance in United States–China joint ventures: A comparative case study, *Academy of Management Journal*, 37: 1478–1517.

Anderson, B. and Dovey, L. (2003) *Wither accountability?* State Services Commission, Wellington. Working paper 18.

Appointments Commission and Department of Health (2003) *Governing the NHS: a guide for NHS boards*. Appointments Commission, London.

Arnetz, J. E. and Arnetz, B. B. (1996) The Development and Application of a Patient Satisfaction Measurement System for Hospital-wide Quality Improvement, *International Journal of Quality in Health Care*, 8(6): 555–66.

Ashby, W. R. (1968) *An introduction to cybernetics*. University Paperback, London.

Audit Commission (2001) *A healthy outlook: local authority oversight and scrutiny of health organistions*. Audit Commission, London.

Audit Commission (2003) *Corporate Governance: Improvement and trust in local public services*. Audit Commission, London.

Ayers, I. and Braithwaite, J. (1992) *Responsive Regulation*. Oxford University Press, Oxford.

Baker, G. R. and Pink, G. H. (1995) A balanced scorecard for Canadian Hospitals, *Healthcare Management Forum*, 8(4): 7–13.

Basle Committee on Banking Supervision (1998) *Framework for internal control systems in banking organisations*. Basle Committee on Banking Supervision, Basle.

Berwick, D. M. (1989) Continuous Improvement as an Ideal in Health Care, *New England Journal of Medicine*, 320: 53–6.

Better regulation task force (2000a) *Alternatives to state regulation*. Better regulation task force, London.

Better regulation task force (2000b) *Principles of good regulation*. Better regulation task force, London.

Better regulation task force (2001) *Annual Report 2000–2001*. Better regulation task force, London.

Better regulation task force (2003) *Imaginative Thinking for Better Regulation*. Better regulation task force London.

Bhagat, S. and Black, B. S. (1999) Uncertain Relationship Between Board Composition and Firm Performance, *Business Lawyer*, 54(3).

Black, J. (1997) *Rule and regulations*. Clarendon Press, Oxford.

Blair, M. M. (1995) *Ownership and control*. The Brookings Institute, Washington DC.

Blair, T. (1996) The Singapore Speech, Singapore.

Bogdanor, V. (1998) *Constitutional Reform in the UK*. Centre for Public Law, University of Cambridge, Cambridge.

Braybrooke, D. and Lindblom, C. E. (1963) *A strategy of decision*. The Free Press, New York.

Brennan, T. and Berwick, D. (1995) *New Rules Regulation, Markets and the Quality of American Health Care*. Jossey-Bass, San Francisco.

Burgess, K., Burton, C. and Parston, G. (2001) *Accountability for results*. Public Service Productivity Panel, London.

Cabinet Office (1999) *Modernising Government*. Cabinet Office, London, Cm 4310.

Cabinet Office (2001) *Better policy making: a guide to regulatory impact assessment*. Cabinet Office, London.

Cabinet Office (2002) *Risk: improving government's capability to handle risk and uncertainty*. Cabinet Office, London.

Cadbury, A. (1993) The corporate governance agenda, *Corporate Governance* pp. 7–15.

Cadbury, A. and The London Stock Exchange (1992) *The financial aspects of corporate governance*. Business Science Press, London.

Caldeira, V. (2000) *Towards and efficient and effective system of internal control and audit of the European Community revenue and expenditure*. Verstehen workshop, Brussels.

Canadian Institute of Chartered Accountants (1997) *Guidance on Assessing Control – the CoCo Principles*. Canadian Institute of Chartered Accountants, Toronto.

Centre for Business Performance (1999) *Implementing Turnbull*. The Institute of Chartered Accountants.

Chapman, C. (2003) Bringing ERM into focus, *Internal Auditor*.

Chen, J., Rathmore, S. S., Radford, M. J. and Krumholz, H. M. (2003) JCAHO Accreditation and Quality of Care for Acute Myocardial Infarction, *Health Affairs*, 22(2).

CIPFA/SOLACE (2001) *Corporate Governance in Local Government*. CIPFA, London.

Clark, W. W. and Bradshaw, T. (2003) *Sustainable Energy in Complex Societies: The Case of the California Energy Crisis*. Elsevier, London.

Clark, W. W. and Demirag, I. (2002) Enron, the Failure of Corporate Governance, *The Journal of Corporate Citizenship*, 8: 105–22.

Clinical governance support team and the national primary and care trust development programme (2003) *The strategic leadership of clinical governance*. Clinical governance support team and the national primary and care trust development programme, Leicester.

Committee of sponsoring organisations – the Treadway Commission (COSO) (1992) *Internal control – integrated framework*. National Commission on fraudulent financial reporting, Washington.

Committee on standards in public life (1996) *Principles of Conduct*. HMSO, London.

Controls Assurance Team (1999) *Guideance on the development and implementation of Controls Assurance for 1999/2000*. NHS Executive, Leeds, annex a.

CoSo (1995) *Internal Control – integrated framework executive summary*. Canadian Institute of Chartered Accountants, Toronto.

Craven, D. W., Piercy, N. F. and Shipp, S. H. (1996) New organisational forms for competing in highly dynamic environments: the network paradigm, *British Journal of Management*, 7: 203–18.

Criteria of control board of the Canadian Institute of Chartered Accountants (1995) *Guidance on control COCO*. Canadian Institute of Chartered Accountants, Toronto.

Culpin, T. (2001) *The Proposed New Law On Corporate Killing*. legalinfowebsite.

Das, T. K. and Teng, B. S. (2001) Trust, Control and Risk in Strategic Alliances: An Integrated Framework, *Organisation Studies* pp. 1–12.

Davies, H. T. O., Nutley, S. M. and Mannion, R. (2000) Organisational culture and quality of health care, *Quality in health care*, 9: 111–19.

Day, P. and Klein, R. (1987) *Accountabilities*. Tavistock, London.

Day, P. and Klein, R. (2004) *The NHS Improvers*. The King's Fund, London.

Deloitte and Touche (2000) *implementing Turnbull – almost 8 months on!* Enterprise risk services, Internet.

Deming, W. (2002) *Out of the crisis*. MIT, Centre for Advanced Engineering Study, Cambridge, Mass.

Department of Health (2000) *The Vital Connection: an equalities framework for the NHS*. Department of Health, London.

Department of Health (2001a) *Building a safer NHS for patients*. The Stationery Office, London.

Department of Health (2001b) *Code of Conduct Code of Accountability*. Department of Health, London.

Department of Health (2001c) *Controls Assurance Project – Guidance First Principles*. Department of Health, London.

Department of Health (2002a) *Assurance: the Board Agenda*. The Department of Health, London.

Department of Health (2002b) *Learning from Bristol:The DH Response to the Report of the Public Inquiry into children's heart surgery at the Bristol Royal Infirmary 1984–1995*. Department of Health, London.

Department of Health (2004) *Standards for better health*. Department of Health, London.

Dewar, S. (2003) *Government and the NHS: Time for a new relationship?* King's Fund, London.

Donabedian, A. (1980) *Explorations in quality assessment and monitoring*. Health Administration Press, Ann Arbor.

Donabedian, A. (1986) Criteria and standards for quality assessment and monitoring, *Quality Review Bulletin*, March: 99–108.

Donabedian, A. (1988a) Quality Assessment and Assurance: unity of purpose, diversity of means, *Inquiry*, 25: 173–92.

Donabedian, A. (1988b) The quality of care: how can it be assessed?, *Journal of the American Medical Association*, 260: 1743–48.

Donabedian, A. (1989) Institutional and professonal responsibilities in quality assurance, *Quality Assurance in health care*, 1(1): 3–11.

Donabedian, A. (1990) The Seven Pillars of Quality, *Archive of Pathology Laboratory Medicine*, 114: 1115–8.

Donaldson, T. and Preston, L. E. (1995) The stakeholder theory of the corporation: Concepts, evidence, and implications, *Academy of Management Review*, 20: 65–91.

Easterbrook, F. H. and Fischel, D. R. (1996) *The Economic Structure of Corporate Law*. Harvard University Press, Boston, Mass.

Economist (2002) The Real Scandal, *Economist*, vol.19: January.

Eisenberg, J. (1997) *Testimony on Health Care Quality*. Before the House Sub-committee on Health and the Environment, USA.

Eisenhardt, K. (1985) Control: Organizational and economic approaches, *Management Science*, 31: 134–49.

encycogov.com. (2004) What is corporate governance? www.encycogov.com.

Fama, E. F. and Jensen, M. C. (2000) Separation of ownership and control, *Journal of Law and Economics*, xxvi: 301–25.

Final Report Joint Committee on Corporate Governance (2001) *Beyond compliance: building a governance culture*. Chartered Accountants of Canada, Toronto.

Finkelstein, S. and Hambrick, D. (1996) *Strategic leadership – top executives and their effects on organisations*. West Publishing, Minneapolis.

Franks, J. and Mayer, C. (1997) Corporate Ownership and Control in the U.K., Germany and France, *Bank of America Journal of Applied Corporate Governance*, 9(4): 30–45.

Friedman, M. (1970) The social responsibility of business is to increase its profits, *New York Times Magazine*, 13: 33.

Friends of the Earth (2001) *Corporate accountability versus corporate responsibility and the Johannesburg Earth Summit*. Friends of the Earth, Internet.

Gaba, D. M. (2000) Structural and organisational issues in patient safety: a comparison of health care to other high-hazard organisations, *California Management Review*, 43(83): 102.

Gamble, A. and Kelly, G. (2001) Shareholder value and the Stakeholder Debate in the UK, *Corporate Governance*, 9(2).

Garrod, N. (1996) *Environmental contingencies and sustainable modes of corporate governance*. Internet.

Garsten, C. and Grey, A. (2001) *Trust, control and Post-bureaucracy*. Organisation Studies.

Garvey, P. R. and Landowne, Z. F. (2004) Risk Matrix: an approach for identifying, assessing and ranking program risks, *Airforce Journal of Logistics*, XXII(i): 18–21.

Government of Victoria (2000) *The application of risk management principles in public health legislation*. Final report.

Green, S. G. and Welsh, M. A. (1998) Cybernetics and dependence: Reframing the control concept, *Academy of Management Review*, 13: 287–301.

Greenbury Committee (1995) *Directors' Remuneration: Report of a Study Group chaired by Sir Richard Greenbury*. London.

Gronroos, C. (1984) A Service Quality Model and its Marketing Implications, *European Journal of Marketing*, 18: 36–44.

HM Treasury (1997) *The Green Book: Appraisal and Evaluation in Central Government*. HM Treasury, London.

HM Treasury (2000a) *Corporate Governance: Statement on internal control*. DAO(GEN)13/'00.

HM Treasury (2000b) *Management of Risk: a strategic overview The Orange Book*, HM Treasury, London.

HM Treasury (2001) *Management of Risk: a strategic overview*. HM Treasury, London.

HM Treasury (2002a) *Audit and Accountability in Central Government. The Government's response to Lord Sharman's report*. HM Treasury, London.

HM Treasury (2002b) *Better regulation task force report on local delivery of central policy: government response*. HM Treasury, London.

Hadorn, D. C. (1991) Setting Health Care Priorities in Oregon, *Journal of the American Medical Association*, 265(17): 2218–25.

Halligan, A. and Donaldson, L. (2001) Implementing clincial governance, *British Medical Journal*, 322: 1413–17.

Hampel Committee report (1998) *Committee on corporate governance: Final Report*. The Stock Exchange, London.

Handy, C. (1994) *The age of paradox*. Penguin, London.

Harrington, A. (2002) *Factors beyond regulatory control*. www.financialdirector.co.uk/Features/1131737).

Harrison, J. J. H. (1998) Corporate governance in the NHS – an assessment of boardroom practice, 6: 140–50.

Hart, O. and Moore, J. (1990) Property rights and the nature of the firm, *Journal of Political Economy*, 98: 1119–58.

Health care standards unit and the risk management working group (2004) *Making it work: guidance on designing and using a risk matrix*. Health care standards unit, Keele.

Health Resources and Services Administration (2000) *Eliminating Health Disparities in the United States*. Rockville, Maryland USA.

Heracleous, L. (2001) What is the impact of corporate governance on organisational performance?, *Corporate Governance*, 9: 165–73.

Higgs, D. (2003) *Review of the Role and Effectiveness of Non-executive Directors*. Department of Trade and Industry, London.

Hirschman, A. O. (1970) *Exit, voice and loyalty*. Harvard University Press, Harvard.

Hood, C., James, O. and Scott, C. (2003) *Regulating government in a 'managerial age': towards a cross-national perspective*. Centre for Analysis of Risk and Regulation, London School of Economics, London.

Hood, C., James, O., Scott, C. and Travers, T. (1998) Regulation inside Government: where new public management meets the audit explosion, *Public Money and Management*, vol. April–June.

Hood, C., James, O., Scott, C. and Travers, T. (1999) *Regulation inside government: waste watchers, quality police and sleaze-busters*. Oxford Unversity Press, Oxford.

House of Commons (1999) *Environment, Transport and Regional Affairs Committeee tenth report*. London.

Houses of the Oireachtais (2002) Waiting Lists: a comparative overview, Parliament of Ireland.

Interdepartmental group on risk assessment (2002) *The Precautionary Principle: Policy and Application*. Health and Safety Executive, London.

Interdepartmental Liaison Group on Risk Assessment (1998) *Improving policy and practice within government departments*. Health and Safety Executive, London, Second Report.

International Organisation of Supreme Audit Institutions (2001) *Internal control: providing a foundation for accountability in Goverment*, Internet.

Jacobs, C. M., Chritoffel, T. H. and Dixon, N. (1976) *Measuring the quality of patient care*, quoted in Brennan and Berwick edn, Ballinger, New York.

Joint Committee on Corporate Governance (2001) *Beyond compliance: building a governance culture*. Chartered Accountants of Canada.

Jun, M., Peterson, R. and Zsidisin, G. A. (1998) The Identification and Measurement of Quality Dimensions in Health Care: focus group interview results, *Health Care Management Review*, 23(4): 81.

Kay, J. (1997) A stakeholding society – what does it mean for business?, *Scottish Journal of Political Economy*, 44(4) 425–36.

King's Fund (2002) *The Future of the NHSA Framework for Debate*. King's Fund, London.

Klein, R. and Day, P. (1989) *Accountabilities in Five Public Services*. Open University Press.

Kohn, L., Corrigan, J. and Donaldson, M. (2000) *To Err is Human: Building a Safer Health System*. National Academy Press, Washington DC.

Kouzes, J. M. and Posner, B. Z. (1999) *Leadership Challenge*. Jossey-Bass, New York.

Le Guen, J. (1999) *Reducing risks, protecting people*. Health and Safety Executive, London.

Lea, R. and Mayo, E. (2002) *The Mutual Health Service*. Institute of Directors and New Economics Foundation, London.

Leape, L. L. (1994) Error in Medicine, *Journal of the American Medical Association*, 272: 1851–7.

Leape, L., Woods, D., Hatlie, M. J., Kizer, K. W. and Schroeder, S. (1998) Promoting patient safety by preventing medical error, *Journal of the American Medical Association*, 280(16): 1–10.

Liefer, R. and Mills, P. K. (1996) An information processing approach for deciding upon control strategies and reducing control loss in emerging organizations, *Journal of Management*, 22: 113–17.

London Stock Exchange (1998) *Combined code for corporate governance*. London Stock Exchange, London.

Lord Irvine of Lairg (1999) *Britain's programme of constitutional change*. University of Leiden, The Netherlands.

Lord Nolan and his committee (1995) *First report of the committee on standards in public life*. HMSO, London.

Lord Sharman (2002) *Holding to Account*. HM Treasury, London.

Mackay, I. L. and Sweeting, R. C. (2000) Perspectives on Integrated Business Risk Management and the Implications for Corporate Governance, *Corporate Governance*, 8(4) 367–74.

Majone, G. (1983) *The Uncertain Logic of Standard Setting*. International Institute for Applied Systems Analysis, Lazenburg, Austria.

March, J. G. a. Z. S. (1987) Managerial Perspectives on Risk and Risk Taking, *Management Science*, 33(11): 1404–18.

McNamee, D. (1996) *Control and Risk Self Assessment*. Mc^2 Management Consulting.

Miller, K. D. (1992) A Framework for Integrated Risk Management in International Business, *Journal of International Business Studies*, 23(2) 311–32.

Millstein, I. M. and MacAvoy, P. W. (1998) The active board of directors and performance of the large publicly traded corporations, *Colombia Law Review*, 98(5).

Ministry of Commerce New Zealand (1999) *A guide to preparing regulatory impact statements*.

Minnow, N. (2002) Terry Savage talks to Nell Minnow, *Chicago Sun Times*, July.

Mitra, S. and Rana, V. (1999) *Children and the Internet: An experiment with minimally invasive education in India*. CSI communications, India.

Monks, R. and Minow, N. (1994) *Corporate Governance*. Blackwell.

Montgomery, C. L. (1993) *Healing through Communication*. Sage, Newbury Park.

Moore, J. D. Jr. (1999) JCAHO drops a survey rating: board says 'commendation award has several weaknesses', *Modern Healthcare*, 29(46).

Morley, S. (2004) *Redefining control: applying complexity theory to corporate governance*. London School of Economics, London.

National Audit Office (2000) *Supporting innovation: managing risk in Government Departments*. National Audit Office, London.

National Audit Office (2001a) *Joining up to improve public services*. National Audit Office, London.

National Audit Office (2001b) *Better regulation: making good use of regulatory impact assessments*. National Audit Office, London.

National Audit Office (2001c) *Modern Policy Making*. National Audit Office, London.

National Audit Office (2002) *2000–2001 General Report of the Comptroller and Auditor General*. National Audit Office, London, HC 335-XIX.

National Audit Office (2004) *Increased resources to improve public services*. National Audit Office, London, (HC 234 2003–2004).

National Consumer Council (1999) *Models of Self Regulation.*

National Expert Advisory Group on safety and quality in Australian health care (1999) *Implementing safety and quality enhancement in health care.* Department of Health and Aged Care, Canberra, First report to Health Ministers.

NHS Executive (1998) *Corporate Governance in the NHS: Controls Assurance Statements 1998/1999 and 1999/2000.* HSC 1998/070.

NHS Executive (1999a) *Governance in the New NHS.* Department of Health, London, HSC 1999/123.

NHS Executive (1999b) *Clinical Governance: in the new NHS.* HSC 1999/065.

O'Neill, O. (2002) *A Question of Trust.* BBC Reith Lecture, London.

OECD (2002) *OECD principles of corporate governance.* Organisations for Economic Co-operation and Development, Paris.

OECD (2003) *Survey of corporate governance developments in OECD countries.*

Office of Government Commerce (2002) *Management of Risk: guidance for practitioners.*

Office of the Deputy Prime Minister (2003) *Delivering proportionate and co-ordinated inspections and audit of authority services.* London.

Office of the Inspector General (OIG) (1999) *The External Review of Hospital Quality, A Call for Greater Accountability.* Office of the Inspector General (OIG), Washington.

Ouchi, W. (1979) A Conceptual Framework for the Design of Organizational Control Mechanism, *Management Science,* 25: 833–48.

Parasuraman, A., Zeithamel, V. A. and Berry, L. L. (1985) A conceptual model of service quality and its implications for future research, *Journal of Marketing,* 49: 41–50.

Parkinson, J. and Kelly, G. (1999) The Combined Code on corporate governance, *The Political Quarterly* pp. 101–7.

Patterson J. (1999) *The Patterson Report – the link between corporate governance and performance.* The Corporate Library, website.

Performance and Innovation Unit (2000) *Wiring it up.* Cabinet Office, London.

Performance and Innovation Unit (2001a) *Strengthening leadership in the public sector.* Performance and Innovation Unit, London.

Performance and Innovation Unit (2001b) *Cabinet Office.* Cabinet Office, London.

Performance and Innovation Unit (2001c) *Better policy delivery and design: a discussion paper.*

Performance and Innovation Unit (2002) *Performance and innovation unit project: risk and uncertainty.* Performance and Innovation Unit, London.

Perry 6 (1997) *Holistic Government.* Demos, London.

Peters, T. and Waterman, R. (1982) *In Search of Excellence.* Harper & Row, New York.

Petts, Horlick-Jones and Murdoch (2001) *Social amplification of risk.* Health and Safety Executive, Caerphilly.

Porter, M. (1990) *Competitive Advantage.* The Free Press, New York.

Powell, D. and Leiss, W. (1997) *Mad cows and mother's milk: The perils of poor risk communication*. McGill-Queen's University Press, Montreal, Canada.

Power, M. (1997) *The audit society: rituals of verification*. Oxford University Press, Oxford.

Public Accounts Committee (1999) *The UK Passport Agency: the passport delays of summer 1999*. House of Commons, London.

Public Accounts Committee (2001) *Managing risk in government departments – First report*. House of Commons, London.

Public Accounts Committee (2002) *Ensuring that policies deliver value for money 49th report*. UK Parliament, London.

Public Audit Forum (2000) *What public sector bodies can expect from their Auditors*. Public Audit Forum, London.

Public Audit Forum (2001) *Propriety and Audit in the Public Sector*. Public Audit Forum, London.

Public Audit Forum (2002) *The Different Roles of External Audit, Inspection and Regulation*. Public Audit Forum, London.

QUEST (2000) *Developing risk management in Department for Culture, Media and Sport sponsored bodies*. Department for Culture Media and Sport, London.

Reeves, C. L. (2000) *Governance in the NHS: letter to Chief Executives*.

Reeves, C. L. (2001) *Organisational Controls Assurance 2000/01: Audit Opinion*.

Report of the ADM working group on risk management (2000) *Risk Management for Canadians*.

Richter, F. J. (1994) The emergence of corporate alliance networks – conversion to self-organisation, *Human systems management*, 13: 16–19.

Roberts, H. and Philip, I. (1996) Prioritising Performance Measures for Geriatric Medical Services: what do patients and providers think?, *Age and Aging*, 25(4): 326.

Roberts, K. H. (1990) Managing High Reliability Organisations, *California Management Review*, 32: 101–13.

Rosenbaum, S. and Teitelbaum, J. D. (2000) Coverage Decisions Versus the Quality of Care: An Analysis of Recent ERISA Judicial Decisions and Their Implications for Employer-Insured Individuals, prepared for the Substance Abuse and Mental Health Services Administration, Washington, USA.

ROSPA (2000) *Occupational Safety Comments on the Government's proposals for reforming the law of involuntary manslaughter*. ROSPA, London.

Rt Hon Alan Milburn MP, S. o. S. f. H. t. t. N. H. N. (2002) *Redefining the National Health Service*. Speech.

Scally, G. and Donaldson, L. (1998) Clinical Governance and the Drive for Quality Improvement in the New NHS in England, *British Medical Journal*, 317: 61–5.

Scott, A. (2000) The Role of Concordats in the New Governance of Britain: Taking Subsidiarity Seriously?, Harvard Law School, Cambridge, MA 02138.

Scrivens, E. (1995) *Accreditation: Protecting the Professional or the Consumer?* Open University Press, Buckingham.

Scrivens, E. (2004) Information for good governance in M. Rigby (ed.) *Vision and Value in Health Information*. Radcliffe Medical Press Ltd, Oxford, pp. 79–90.

Sheen, M. J. (1987) *MV Herald of Free Enterprise. Report of Court No. 8074 Formal Investigation*. Department of Transport, London.

Simon, H. A. (1991) Organizations and Markets, *Journal of Economic Perspectives*, 5(2): 25–44.

Sir John Bourn (2002) *Reinforcing Positive Approaches to Risk Management in Government*. Institute of Risk Management, London.

Sir William Beveridge (1942) *Social Insurance and Allied Services*. HMSO London.

Sitkin, S. and Roth, N. (1993) Explaining the limited effectiveness of legalistic 'remedies' for trust/distrust, *Organization Science*, 4: 367–92.

Slovic, P. (2002) *Perception of Risk Posed by Extreme Events*. Conference paper, New York, Risk Management Strategies in an uncertain world.

Spangenberg, S. (2001) The Political Economy of a British Stakeholder Society, *Briefing notes in economics*, 47: 1–12.

Standards Australia (1999) *Australia/New Zealand Standard 4360 Risk Management*. Standards Australia, Sydney.

Standards Australia (2000) *Key risks facing Australian organisations*. Standards Australia, Sydney.

Steinberg, R. M. (1993) Internal control – integrated framework: a landmark study, *The CPA Journal On line*.

Strategic policy making team, Cabinet office (1999) *Professional policy making in the twenty-first century*. Cabinet Office, London.

Strategy Unit (2002) *Creating Public Value: An analytical framework for public service reform*. Cabinet Office, London.

Sydow, J. (1998) Understanding the constitution of interorganizational trust in C. Lane and R. E. Bachmann (eds). *Trust within and between organisations, conceptual issues and empirical applications*. Oxford University Press, Oxford, pp. 31–63.

Taylor, K., Plowman, R. and Roberts, J. (2001) *The Challenge of Hospital Acquired Infection*. The Stationery Office, London.

The Amazing Disintegrating Firm (2001) Economist, *Economist*, vol. 6 December.

The Canadian Institute of Chartered Accountants (1995) *Guidance on Control*, Toronto.

The Canadian Institute of Chartered Accountants (1999) *Guidance for Directors: dealing with risk in the boardroom*. Toronto.

The Canadian Institute of Chartered Accountants (2003) *Guidance on assessing control*. Toronto.

The consumer consortium on assisted living newsletter (2000) *Deemed Status*. Consumer consortium on assisted living, summer.

The Internal Control Working Party of the Institute of Chartered Accountants in England and Wales (1999) *Internal Control: Guidance for Directors on the Combined Code: The Turnbull Report*. Institute of Chartered Accountants, London.

The King Committee (2001) *King Report on Corporate Governance for South Africa – draft for public comment.* Institute of Directors, Parktown, South Africa.

The Presidential/Congressional Commission on Risk Assessment and Risk Management (1997) *Risk assessment and risk management in decision making.* The Presidential/Congressional Commission on Risk Assessment and Risk Management, Washington.

The Prime Minister's Office of Public Services Reform (2002) *Reforming our public services: principles into practice.* London.

The Report of the Public Inquiry into children's heart surgery at the Bristol Royal Infirmary 1984–1995 (2001) *Learning from Bristol.* The Stationery Office, London.

Treadway Report (1987) *Report on the National Commission on Fraudulent Reporting.* National Commission on Fraudulent Reporting, Washington.

Treasury Board of Canada (1999) *Planning, Reporting and Accountability Structures.* Treasury Board of Canada, Ottawa.

Treasury Board of Canada (2000) *Integrated Risk Management Framework.* Treasury Board of Canada, Ottawa.

Tricker, R. I. (1984) *Corporate Governance.* Gower Press, Aldershot.

Tricker, R. L. (1994) *International Corporate Governance.* Simon and Shuster, Singapore.

Trubeck, D. M. and Mosher, J. S. (2001) *New Governance, EU Employment Policy and the European Social Market.* Jean Monnet Center, New York University School of Law.

Turnbull, N. (1999) *Guidance for Directors.* Institute of Chartered Accountants, London.

Turnbull, S. (1997) Corporate Governance: its scope, concerns and theories, *Corporate Governance,* 5(4): 180–205.

Turnbull, S. (2003) *Why audits fail.* The corporate library, Internet.

Vass, P. and Simmonds, G. (2001a) *External Review Second 'Updated' Overview Report.* Public Services Productivity Panel, London.

Vass, P. and Simmonds, G. (2001b) *External Review Second 'Updated' Overview Report: background research findings.* Public Services Productivity Panel, London.

Vladeck, B. (1988) Quality Assurance through External Controls, *Inquiry,* vol. Spring, pp. 100–7.

Walsh, K. R. and Schneider, H. (2002) *The role of motivation and risk behaviour in software development success,* (7th edn).

Weiner, B. J. and Alexander, J. A. (1993) Hospital governance and quality of care: a critical review of transitional roles, *Medical Care Research and Review,* 50(4) 375–411.

Wheeler, D. and Silanpaa, M. (1997) *The Stakeholder Corporation.* Pitman Publishing, London.

Wilde, K., Jones, P. and Scrivens, E. (2004) *Discussion on the use of controls assurance self-assessment data.* Health Care Standards Unit, Keele.

Williamson, J. W., Goldschmidt, P. G. and Jilson, I. A. (1979) *Medical Practice Information Demonstration Project: Final Report*. Office of the Assistance Secretary of Health, DHEW, Baltimore.

Working group on harmonisation of risk assessment procedures in the scientific committees advising the European Commission in the area of human and environmental health (2000) *First report on the harmonisation of risk assessment procedures – part one*. European Commission, Internet.

World Health Organisation Secretariat (2001) *Quality of patient care: patient safety*. WHO, Geneva.

Yataganas, X. (2001) *Delegation of regulatory authority in the European Union*. Paper presented at a hearing organized by the European Governance task force in Brussels on 12 March 2001, Brussels.

Index

Page numbers in *italics* refer to tables and figures.

Related books from Open University Press
Purchase from www.openup.co.uk or through your local bookseller

GOVERNING MEDICINE
Theory and Practice

Andrew Gray and Stephen Harrison

Gray and Harrison have assembled an impressive array of authors to analyse the changing role of the medical profession. The contributions range from historical analyses of the relationship between government and doctors, to detailed examination of the implementation of clinical governance in the NHS. All offer important insights into an issue that lies at the heart of contemporary debates in health policy.

Chris Ham, University of Birmingham

This book brings together the most pertinent discussion on clinical governance by some of the most eminent practitioners and researchers in the United Kingdom. Since New Labour's institution of clinical governance through its White Paper in 1997, there has been a good deal of debate about the history, theory and practice of Clinical Governance and the governance of clinical care.

Divided into three parts, the book contains sections on:

- Medicine, Autonomy and Governance
- Evidence, Science and Medicine
- Realizing Clinical Governance

Starting with the differing definitions of the term clinical governance, the contributors discuss the relationship of medicine and governance, the challenges that evidence-based medicine makes upon clinical practice and move on to suggest possible futures for clinical governance.

Written by a team of experienced academics and practitioners, this book is aimed at reflective health professionals, as well as students and academics in the fields of health policy, health services management, social policy and public policy.

Contributors
Marian Barnes, Andy Bilson, David Byrne, Barbara Coyle, Pieter Degeling, Tracy Finch, Rob Flynn, Andrew Gray, Steve Harrison, Rick Iedema, John Kennedy, Fergus Macbeth, Frances Mair, Sharyn Maxwell, Carl May, Michael Moran, Maggie Mort, Nancy Redfern, Chandra Vanu Som, Jane Stewart, Barbara Telfer, Stephen Watkins, Sue White.

Contents
Governing Medicine: An Introduction – **PART 1: MEDICINE, AUTONOMY AND GOVERNANCE** – 'Soft Bureaucracy', Governmentality and Clinical Governance: Theoretical Approaches to Emergent Policy – Governing Doctors in the British Regulatory State – Medicine and Government: Partnership Spurned? – Medicine and Management: Autonomy and Authority in the National Health Service – Practitioner Perspectives on Objectives and Outcomes of Clinical Governance: Some Evidence from Wales – **PART 2: EVIDENCE, SCIENCE AND MEDICINE** - Evidence-Based: What Constitutes Valid Evidence? – Limits of Governance: Interrogating the Tacit Dimensions of Clinical Practice – Telemedicine and Clinical Governance: Controlling Technology, Containing Knowledge – Affect, Anecdote and Diverse Debates: User Challenges to Scientific Rationality – **PART 3: REALIZING CLINICAL GOVERNANCE** - What Counts is What Works: Postgraduate Medical Education and Clinical Governance – Developing the Human Resource Dimension of Clinical Governance – Restructuring Clinical Governance to Maximize its Developmental Potential – Governing Medicine: Governance, Science and Practice – References – Index.

224pp 0 335 21435 5 (Paperback) 0 335 21436 3 (Hardback)

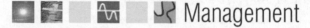
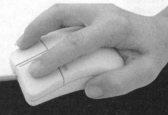